DESTINATIC

A bookful of uncommon sense.
Eden Fruitarianism Explained

FIRST EDITION - September 2013

ISBN: 978-1-291-54086-4 (Paperback)
ISBN: 978-1-326-07814-0 (Ebook)

Author: Mango Wodzak
Illustrations: Mango Wodzak
Cover Photos: Květoslava Martincova
Cover Design: Mango Wodzak
Author Website: http://www.fruitnut.net - Home of Eden Fruitarianism
Publisher: http://www.lulu.com

Both the e-version and the printed version of my books are available to
buy here:

http://www.lulu.com/spotlight/DestinationEden

Enjoyed this book? Please like the Facebook Page:

https://www.facebook.com/EdenFruitarianism/

If you wish to bulk buy this book (ten or more), to sell through your
business, or at appropriate venues, or simply to give away as presents,
send me a private message through my website or facebook page, and
I will send you a link to a discount price page.

0.55

*"You don't have
to see the
whole staircase
Just take the
FIRST STEP!"*
- Martin Luther King

*"Beautiful things happen
in your life when you
distance yourself
from all that is negative."*
- Unknown

*"The greater the difficulty,
the more glory in surmounting it.
Skilful pilots gain their reputation
from storms and tempests."*
- Epicetus

*"Everything changes when you start
to emit your own frequency rather than
absorbing the frequencies around you,
when you start imprinting your intent
on the universe rather than receiving
an imprint from existence."*
- Barbara Marciniak

55

Table of Contents

SECTION FOUR – Additional Related Thoughts 197

SECTION ZERO

*"A very great vision is needed
and the man who has it
must follow it as the eagle
seeks the deepest blue of the sky."*
- Crazy Horse
(Oglala Lakota Sioux (circa 1840-1877))

*"He who would do great things should
not attempt them all alone."*
- Seneca proverb

*"You're off to Great Places!
Today is your day!
Your mountain is waiting,
So... get on your way!"*
- Dr. Seuss

ACKNOWLEDGEMENTS

My gratitude goes out to my loving partner, Květa, for her feedback and patience with me as I struggled to finish this book, forever tweaking and fine tuning it. Never fully content. I finally realised I likely never will be.

My thanks also goes to Zalan, Konrad and Esther, for their help in proof reading, and initial feedbacks of draft versions.

Finally thanks to everyone else I've met on my journey, who has offered insight and encouragement, and all the great people out there who are ready for the message and vision I'm about to share with you.

DEDICATION

This book is dedicated to the wave of awakening consciousnesses, to those who can see past society indoctrination, and who, looking positively forward to a love and light filled world, are prepared to make the lifestyle changes necessary for such a vision.

Nothing will ever be attempted
if all possible objections
must first be overcome.
- Samuel Johnson

DISCLAIMER

Let it be clear from the onset, that I am neither a doctor nor a qualified nutritional expert. I left school at the tender age of sixteen and am happy to have had no other formal education. Whether or not you choose to share or act on the thoughts and visions I present throughout this book is your personal matter.

I have no desire to take on any obligations for your resulting personal choices. If you are in need of someone to take responsibility for your decisions in life, then I suggest you consult a suitable, accredited professional.

> Who you are and what you experience is based upon the choices you make. It's not your parents, your past relationships, your job, the economy, the book you read, what someone said, the weather, an argument, nor your age, that are to blame (or credit!). You, and only you, are responsible for every decision and choice you make. Period.

My advice within this book is that you follow or do what you truly believe to be correct. That you read my words with an open mind, give them time to digest, and then reach your own conclusions.

Naturally, I cannot deny, I would like for readers to share my vision, but my desires should not interfere with your own judgements. I'm not here to tell you how you yourself should or should not live your life, what you should or should not believe, or how you should or should not eat. These are your choices, and you alone must decide what you feel is right for you.

> "We are all visitors to this time, this place. We are just passing through. Our purpose is to observe, to learn, to grow, to love.. and then we return home."
> - Australian Aboriginal Proverb

The purpose of this book is for me to explain why I have made the choices I have.

Make of it what you will..

Don't be afraid to be open minded,
your brain isn't going to fall out.
- Unknown

PREFACE

By Květa

Lies have corrupted moral values, and through those lies Eden has been lost. Eden has been stolen from us, and our lives stripped of love. To this day, Eden is a fantasy instead of a reality. For most of us Eden does not exist. Puzzled minds delivering confusion and creating pain. Eden is deserted. This is the essence of this book. Mango pinpoints the reasons why.

However, the essence of this book is also joyous. Mango shares his own experiences and a radiant future vision. He hopes to inspire others, and explains how to free all existence from sorrow, embracing instead a happy, love filled life.

Květoslava Martincova - July 2013

By Zalan

Mango's love and life shine brightly throughout this book of sunlight. Refreshing and powerful, a sacred recipe for love, peace, goodwill, and sustainable living. A deeply private, honest and simple account of the journey of his inner child, confronted by violence and suffering, seeking explanations, and modifying his life choices and actions in response.

From an early childhood honed by Monty Python and the Goodies, as a teenage altar boy flirting with reality, science fiction and a creative lifestyle, to an adult struggling to combine ethics and compassion within his social and cultural setting, we now witness the fully developed, integrated, wholistic, spiritual nature of a self professed Eden Fruitarian!

Couched in the genre of 'isms' the novel text is compiled from well-proven experience, with ample portions of reality, research and imagination, from someone with his feet on the ground. A generous lifetime of home grown wisdom, some colourful language, a dash of excitement, a couple of licks of irony, garnished with revelations, and a good sprinkle of fun and humour. Definitely one of the most assimilable books I have read.

Shoes off, step inside, leave your prejudice at the door, settle down in a comfortable chair with a bowl of Mango's fruit salad, and hold on tightly to your essentials, while you join Mango on his flight to fruity freedom; be prepared to gorge the lot.

Life as it is, naked and exposed, our social and cultural norms questioned, while nature's secrets are disclosed; a new bench mark in un-fired un-cooking, with an abundance of ideas that will fire your brain, and a choice of words that will melt in your mouth, this unique tome is serious fun, and funnily serious.

It is an honour to introduce this work, which I consider a major contribution from a brave heart and soul, with the capacity to influence each of us willing to walk the path of personal responsibility while traversing the puddles and slippery slopes of self-awareness. It is very likely your life is *not* here right now. If you are interested in free expression, personal ethics, philosophy, animal rights, health and the challenge of culinary reading, see how you go digesting it slowly, but be prepared to be stimulated. My fingers are still burning from turning the pages.

In documenting his quest for light, Mango has produced a brilliant tale. As self confessed fruit-nuts, he and his partner Květa are without peer. Part of their recent journey to Eden maybe viewed at 'Pure Fruit[1]' on Vimeo. Welcome to Eden Fruitarianism, a seamless trajectory to paradise, and many happy returns!

Zalan Glen - August 2013

*A lie doesn't become truth, wrong doesn't become right, and
evil doesn't become good, just because it is accepted by a majority.*
- Unknown

*"The earth is our mother. Whatever befalls the earth,
befalls the sons and daughters of the earth.
This we know. All things are connected
like the blood which unites one family.
All things are connected.
We did not weave the web of life, we are merely strands in it.
Whatever we do to the web we do to ourselves."*
- Chief Seattle

INTRODUCTION

Hi, my Name's Mango, and I'm a fruitarian.

In claiming to be fruitarian, I don't mean one of the multitude of fruitarians out there who are scared to eat only fruit and advise people that if they do so they will become deficient, get sick, and ultimately die an early, drawn-out, demineralised death. I'm not one of those fruitarians who advise people to make fruit an arbitrary percentage of their diet and then the rest, greens, nuts and seeds. Nor am I one of those fruitarians obsessed with calorie counting, and analysing the handful of separately classified scientific elements purportedly microscopically available within each fruit.

I am also not one of the vast bulk of fruitarians who sully fruits by referring to them degradingly as sugars and fats, nor one whose focus is predominantly on fitness and one's ability and prowess in triathlons or iron-man competitions. Although there are plenty of those kinds of fruitarians out there; I'm not one of them!

> One evening an old Cherokee told his grandson about a battle that goes on inside people. He said: "My son, the battle is between two wolves inside us all. One is Evil - It is anger, envy, jealousy, sorrow, regret, greed, arrogance, self-pity, guilt, resentment, inferiority, lies, false pride, superiority and ego. The other is Good - It is joy, peace, love, hope, serenity, humility, kindness, benevolence, empathy, generosity, truth, compassion and faith."
> The grandson thought about it for a minute and then asked his grandfather: "Which wolf wins?"
> The old Cherokee simply replied: "The one you feed."

I'm currently one of a very rare minority of fruitarians who advocate hundred percent raw, fresh, ripe, fruit, fruitarianism. I differentiate between nuts and fruits, dried, shrivelled fruit and fresh, ripe fruit. I don't believe greens should ultimately form part of one's diet, and I don't drink sugar cane and/or coconut juice.

I believe in practising what I preach. I talk of what I believe to be true fruitarianism, fruitarianism as it is meant to be, the understanding of which also happens to be the key toward (re-)establishing Eden on this planet.

I openly admit that parts of this book are about beliefs, and you will not fail to notice that I actively shun scientific evidence to support these beliefs. So if it happens that you've stumbled upon this book and you're interested in the concept of fruitarianism but are expecting to find pages of nutritional tables coupled with the latest scientific viewpoints to support fruitarianism, then I should come right out and tell you now, that these expectations will definitely not be fulfilled, at least not through this book.

I will not be breaking down foods into their supposed constituent microscopic elements, nor will I be balancing pHs, complimenting [sic] proteins, tracing elements, food combining nor listing recipes. I will however, explain why I actively and consciously eschew such an approach to fruitarianism.

One of many things that appear clear to me, is that the raw food movement has been both commandeered and corrupted by a business-minded minority who quote nutritional science to suit their needs and make it seem as though eating raw is overly complex. By employing a certain amount of tactical scaremongering, they hoodwink the uncomprehending gullible into believing that they must first study hard under the greased palms and guidance of an expert, or attend countless costly seminars. The alternative being to surely succumb to a variety of cleverly christened deficiencies.

> "Many would rather believe a lie, because the truth requires change." - Tony Gaskins

I've read enough books to know that somehow or other, nutritional science can be used to prove many conflicting theories. I believe this is because such research is far from complete, and is therefore open to being interpreted in more than one way. Consequently nutritional science can be easily manipulated and used to convince people of whatever the authors desire. Personally, I find the idea of following a nutritional science, based on a largely incomplete set of facts, to be rather absurd, sadly often so complexly absurd, that it borders on the dangerous. Instead, I believe that when it comes to food, science is a false trail and our one true guideline should be ethics. My belief is that love is the one true force, it alone is responsible in keeping the universe ticking. Once this concept has been fully embraced, the innate intelligence of the body, with its own inner physiological wisdom can alone be fully trusted to guide us toward our true individual nutritional needs at any given moment in time.

> "Time and time again, throughout the history of medical practice, what was once considered as *scientific* eventually becomes regarded as *bad practice*." - David Stewart

Living solely on a fruit diet, following the guidelines of Eden Fruitarianism, does not involve enormous amounts of prior knowledge and long laborious PhD Discourses. This book explains why I believe that to be true.

In case you are at a stage where the supposed facts, figures and statistics of a purportedly proven science seem essential, or should you have already decided that my approach is too ethereal for your own personal liking, then there are plenty of other books for you to choose from. If you would rather hear the opinion of someone who has been indoctrinated and/or has a string of letters after their name, then I suggest you forget this book and look elsewhere. Exercise free will and pass it on to someone who you feel could appreciate it more, or else burn it for fear that the gullible may be corrupted.

EVERY TIME YOU FIND SOME HUMOUR IN A DIFFICULT SITUATION, YOU WIN.

In light of the overall absence of nutritional pseudo-science, I am, however, no less confident in my stance, and by no means suggesting to be taken any less seriously. I merely state this as further means of a disclaimer. Again, whether you agree with my musings is for you alone to decide. I have made my choices and am happy with them; even open to changing them should I ever be compelled enough to do so.

I write both from plenty of experience, and from the overall success of my persistence. Do not expect though, for this book to be solely full of ramblings on food. Rather it is a collection of thoughts, many of which happen to be, by their very nature, food related.

"The truth will set you free. But first it will piss you off." - Gloria Steinem

When this book first began taking form back in the year 2000, I tentatively christened it "Destination Eden - Barefoot Fruitarianism Explained". At the time, I believed that the addition of the word "barefoot" was sufficiently descriptive to distinguish this particular brand of fruitarianism from the ever more popular "I fear fruit" fruitarianism. But over the years, since I began writing, I've noticed that even among the other self-christened fruitarians, there are also those who call themselves barefoot fruitarians. Yet they regularly don flip flops or Vibram Fivefinger shoes, and thus add further confusion to the already chaotic mayhem of non-descriptive titles. Clearly I needed to come up with a better distinguishing word, one that could intelligibly separate the wheat from the chaff. Thus the phrase Eden Fruitarianism was born, and here's to hoping that it too will not fall victim to semantic abuse.

There are times however, where I will still refer to the philosophy in this book as barefoot fruitarianism, or just plain fruitarianism, and at all times will be considering the titles synonymous with the freshly minted Eden Fruitarianism.

"Smiles are contagious. Go forth and contaminate as many people as you can!" - Unknown

The philosophy and lifestyle of Eden Fruitarianism is multi-tiered, and although ultimately not too difficult to grasp, it does require a full understanding of each of its various levels in order to succeed. The purpose of this book is to shed light on each of those levels, with the hope that in doing so, you too may choose to embrace the age old philosophy of fruitarianism.

"Oh, Great Spirit,
whose voice I hear in the winds
and whose breath gives life to all the world, hear me.
I am small and weak.
I need your strength and wisdom.
Let me walk in beauty and make my eyes
ever behold the red and purple sunset.
Make my hands respect the things you have made
and my ears sharp to hear your voice.
Make me wise so that I may understand
the things you have taught my people.
Let me learn the lessons you have hidden
in every leaf and rock.
I seek strength, not to be superior to my brother,
but to fight my greatest enemy - myself.
Make me always ready to come to you
with clean hands and straight eyes,
so when life fades, as the fading sunset,
my spirit will come to you
without shame."
American Indian - Lakota - Chief Yellow Lark - 1887

"One thing to remember is to talk to the animals.
If you do, they will talk back to you.
But if you don't talk to the animals,
they won't talk back to you,
then you won't understand,
and when you don't understand
you will fear, and when you fear
you will destroy the animals,
and if you destroy the animals,
you will destroy yourself."
- Chief Dan George,
(Tsleil-Waututh (1899 - 1981))

"Grown men can learn from
very little children,
for the hearts of the little children are pure.
Therefore, the Great Spirit may show
to them many things which older people miss."
- Black Elk,
(Oglala Lakota Sioux (1863-1950))

"All things share the same breath
- the beast, the tree, the man.
The air shares its spirit
with all the life it supports."
- Chief Seattle

You know the world has gone mad when those who
have enlightened, compassionate views and
future visions, are accused of borderline insanity,
ridiculed and criticised for thinking positively.

SECTION ONE

THE NEED FOR CHANGE
OF CONSUMER HABITS
-Isms Explained

MODERN DAY EVOLUTION

| SHOD OMNIVORE | VEGETARIAN | VEGAN | RAW VEGAN | BAREFOOT FRUITARIAN |

"Our quest, our earth walk, is to look within, to know who we are, to see that we are connected to all things, that there is no separation, only in the mind."
- Lakota Seer

OMNIVORISM

Slippery Slope

I've heard it said by some that marijuana is the first step taken on the road to heavy drugs. It is my belief however, that the first step is taken long before such an eventuality. Long before we taste our first drops of alcohol, or experiment secretively with our first wheeze on a cigarette we are on that road. It's weathered even before we suffer our first coffee, or embark upon the fried crispy boulevard of denatured junk food. The path we are generally set upon from birth leads pretty much inevitably there, sooner or later. The only thing is, we often reach there without ever acknowledging the fact.

> I know a guy who's addicted to brake fluid. He says he can stop whenever he wants.

If it isn't clear already, I'm taking liberties with the definition of heavy drugs, and referring also to the synthetic, chemical based, mind-altering drugs gleefully dispensed by the pharmaceutical industry.

I think it indubitably correct, as the old adage, that goes *humans are creatures of habit*. Indeed, habits can become so ingrained that from our own individual perspectives, we often become simply obliviously unrecognising of their presence.

This is surely the case with certain lifestyle choices that are unwittingly thrust upon us at an early age. Often so young that they, more often than not, remain unnoticed, unquestioned and unchallenged throughout the duration of one's entire earthly existence.

> The Devolution of Shod Omnivorism:
> Eat, drink and be merry.
> Wine, women and song.
> Sex and drugs and rock and roll.
> Blood, sweat and tears.

Let me give an example. We all enter this world as potential barefoot fruitarians. Fruit has that up front mixture of appeals, vibrant colours, the tantalising textures and deliciously sweet flavours that provided corruption and addiction are not already imbued, are instinctively appealing to all children. But alas it's a path few of us are privileged enough, or permitted to embark upon at such an early age. Instead, it rarely takes too long following nascence, before we find ourselves as involuntary shod omnivores. Rarely is such a state of affairs ever cross-examined.

Shod Omnivore

Shod omnivore, you say? Yes, this, I propose, is the antipode of the barefoot fruitarian; the path a vast majority of us are placed upon, and the one the vast majority of us follow until our untimely graves. Rarely also is such a path ever contested, and yet rarer is it forsaken.

Shod Omnivorism; it pretty much sums up the current state of the world. I find the word 'shod' deeply descriptive; it conjures such an archaic barbaric feeling, of being shackled and tamed, captive and downtrodden. Omnivorism is the concept that every living and non-living thing on this planet is a potential meal, and God forbid that anyone should question another's right to eat whatever, whoever[2] and however they desire. Shod and Omnivorism together truly emphasise the sad disequilibrium of the dominant prevailing human mindset.

One thing consumed drugs all have in common, is our initial natural aversion toward them. The first mouthful of alcohol we drink is generally followed by an involuntary grimace. The first puff on a chemical-laden cigarette is followed often by a cough and splutter as the body tries to repel the alien pollution thrust upon it. Our first coffee and tea are generally also greeted somewhat similarly. Of course, it is frequently the case that despite these initial reactions, we push on past them until addiction is formed. Cooked food, although noticeably less recognised as addictive, evokes no less an initial reaction. Think of all those babies whose faces screw up in displeasure vainly attempting rejection of the denatured slop thrust upon them, and the hours spent crying from stomach pains. By the time they are advanced enough to linguistically voice their lack of desire for such foods, they are, alas, already well hooked.

Unlike other omnivores that basically eat their food as nature provides,

> "I braced myself to watch my first murder, I had taken the first sedative in my life an hour earlier, it seemed to get me through. When the cow is locked in the stun box she looks upwards and a captive bolt pistol is aimed at her head. A steel shaft 7cms long penetrates her skull and renders her unconscious. It can take several attempts to hit the right spot. This happened and the cow desperately kept trying to avoid the gun by banging and clanging her body into the sides of the stun pen. Our eyes met just as the bolt entered her head. My life is frozen in that moment and I promised her that for the rest of my life I would do all I could to shut down abattoirs. The blood stained notes are still in my files."
> - Confessions of a slaughterhouse inspector

the shod omnivore looks at anything as being a potential meal. We start off our days with cooked cornflakes covered in cooked (pasteurised) milk, or greasy fried bread with birds' eggs and thinly sliced pig belly flesh. For lunch it's pulverised baked wheat with cooked pasty spreads smeared on top, and for dinner, fired animal fleshes with potatoes. Not only do we make a habit of all this, but we go about telling everyone how healthy it is too!

Thus it is highly likely that this sad disequilibrium of which I speak, will be altogether lost and unclear to many, like spraying perfume on a pig; hence here I sit now, attempting to clarify the reasoning behind my conclusions. Hopefully after reading through this book, light may be shed, and who knows, the proverbial truffula seed (made illustrious through the words of Dr. Seuss in his book *The Lorax*[3]; my all time favourite children's book) may be sown.

> This girl said she recognised me from the vegan club, but I'd never seen herbivore.

I am an optimist, and at least some of the seeds disseminated will surely fall on fertile soil, take root, and sprout.

Read on!

"The food you eat can either be the safest
and most powerful form of medicine,
or the slowest form of poison"
- Ann Wigmore

Nothing will be "rammed down your throat"
in this book; you are reading voluntarily.

"McDonalds announced it's considering a more humane way of slaughtering its animals. You know they fatten them up and then kill them. You know the same thing they do to their customers, isn't it?"
- Comedian Jay Leno

VEGETARIANISM

At some point in the past, I temporarily hypothesised that the reason why the world was not predominantly vegetarian was essentially a question of intelligence. Indeed, a two decade study that began back in the 1970s, which had over 8,000 participants, seemed to indicate a correlation between higher intelligence and vegetarianism[4]. However, not knowing all details, or factors present, I think it a little unwise to jump immediately to conclusions.

On life's path, I have encountered numerous flesh-eaters of strikingly high intelligence, who have apparently never stopped to consider the

> If vegetarians eat vegetables, what do humanitarians eat?

consequences of their omnivorism. This initially lead me to believe that the missing factor was more one of ignorance than intelligence.

It seemed a logical assumption, but with time it became pretty obvious, that even when faced with the blatant facts, most people, regardless of their IQ level, are still unable to see any need to rethink their consumer habits.

This made me delve further, to reconsider possible reasons for this apparent failing of humanity. Clearly there must be another missing ingredient, something else that humans are lacking. I believe that missing ingredient to be empathy.

Empathy

There comes a time when everyone should seriously empathise.

Wikipedia defines *empathy* as "the capacity to recognise feelings that are being experienced by another sentient or semi-sentient being". Empathy is a prerequisite for experiencing

EMPATHISE!

compassion, and compassion is precisely what this world is most in need of. It's the crucial emotion required to help free the world from the thralls of depravity in which it finds itself ensnared [5] [6].

Actually, in retrospect, it's a good thing that compassion relies on empathy rather than intelligence. We are all capable of compassion, regardless of where we intellectually stand! Intellectually, many people know roughly what goes on behind closed slaughterhouse doors, but even though there is a vague surface knowledge, on a deeper level they really don't see what is happening.

In general, we have a very strange relationship with species other than our own. We may selectively nurture feelings and form relationship with particular animals, fully acknowledging their uniqueness in the process. Bonds are often formed which make it unthinkable for someone to harm their chosen animal friend. Cats and dogs are prime examples of animals that humans regularly become attached to. They are taken in as members of the family and to a lesser (or greater!) extent, are treated as such.

> "If you were alone on a deserted island with a pig, would you eat the pig or starve to death?"
>
> "Hmm. If you were not alone, and living on a planet with seven billion people, had access to unlimited fresh fruits, vegetables, nuts, beans, and other healthy foods, and knew animals suffer and die horrible deaths, so you could eat them, when you don't need to eat them to survive, would you continue to eat them?"
>
> The difference between our questions is that your scenario will never happen and mine is the choice you face right now. Which do you believe is worth answering? - Andrew Kirschner

Being an alien observer, one might think that forming such attachments would help humans to have a better understanding of the uniqueness of each and every individual animal, regardless of species. Yet for some reason, the majority of us are seemingly unable to think outside the narrow box we were placed into. We may see the distinctiveness of a dog's personality, and appreciate that the dog is in many ways similar to ourselves; in need of companionship, affection and other general life comforts and necessities. We may see and relate to the sadness of the dog when he is unfairly treated, abused and/or malnourished. Indeed, we have even established organisations that have made it unlawful to treat such animals unjustly.

> Choose Empathy over Apathy!

In moving away from the few chosen species, an altogether different story is revealed. Take the pig, for example, which in many ways is quite similar to a dog. Indeed, by some accounts, they are said to be of a higher intelligence than dogs. The minority of people who have nurtured a relationship with one, can testify as to how they can be equally loyal and faithful as any dog. They can be just as playful, just as humorous, just as protective, just as loving.

Similarly to dogs and ourselves, pigs will do their utmost to avoid both intentional and unintentional harm to themselves, as well as others they have formed attachments to. They will cry when cold, fearful, lonely, or suffering in pain. And yet, generally the only place they receive in our hearts is one of being added artery fat. In contrast to appearing wide eyed *at* the breakfast table, waiting to be petted and treated, they appear *on* the breakfast table, with their eyes removed and their bodies bloodily butchered into rashes.

> "Compassion, in which all ethics must take root, can only attain its full breadth and depth if it embraces all living creatures and does not limit itself to mankind."
> - Albert Schweitzer

In order to satisfy the appetite of the masses, the life of a western pig is filled with far more suffering and cruelty than the likes of that which the RSPCA would ever permit if the victim were a cat or dog. This is a harsh truth that the majority of us are unwilling to face and the reason why time needs to be set aside to practise empathy.

Just why there is this blatant discrimination against pigs and other animals bred for consumption, is altogether unclear. On the one hand we attempt to instil a sense of moral and justice into our children in regards to other animal species; that we should treat them with dignity and respect. While on the other hand, there is this generally accepted attitude of "animals are ours to do with as we please".

> "You are not responsible for the programming you picked up in childhood. However, as an adult, you are 100% responsible for fixing it." - Unknown

By way of demonstration, children may be taken to local parks where they are good-naturedly, yet ignorantly, taught to feed the ducks stale white bread, while generally being told to keep their distance and respect their space. Meanwhile, back at home we are taught how to fry the wings of chickens (and ducks!), and even how cows' bottoms should best be tenderised and seasoned, while the ribs of a pig with a violently bloody history, sit fully disrespected festering in the microwave. This is a sort of moral schizophrenia known in psychology as:

Cognitive Dissonance

Cognitive dissonance[7], discomfort experienced when simultaneously holding two or more opposing beliefs, is the reason why meat eaters get so embarrassed, anxious, flustered and often irrational when these conflicting values are pointed out to them. Make it a cat's bottom, the ribs of a dog and the pale tender flesh of young puppies, and people will become furious! I've seen cases on the Internet, of a dog being locked in a car for several hours and comments from people so enraged, that they threaten physical violence toward the perpetrator; some even crying out for the owners to be faced with the death penalty! These self same people will likely not think twice about the animals on their plates. In fact, they usually react more strongly toward such events (dogs locked in cars) than do most vegans. The often unconsidered, deep seated reasoning behind their indignation, is to draw away attention from their own wrong doings toward animals, and focus it elsewhere. If they shout loud enough, perhaps people won't notice that they themselves, are behind far worse animal treatment!

> "We say we want a loving world, a peaceful world, but we cannot cultivate that love if negative vibes get into us. One way we can bring negative vibrations is through our food. That is why food should come to us as an offering of love. Whatever we eat should be the product of love. When I say a love offering, I do not mean that someone cooks a nice chicken soup or broiled steak and then offers it to you lovingly. The question is, "Did the animal who died to make that steak love you?" I do not think any animal would lovingly die for you. Will a cow come and say, "Oh you seem to be very weak and hungry, would you like my thigh for your soup? Take it." No, you have to kill it, destroy it. In the same way when you catch a fish, it does not come willingly. You have to cheat the fish by throwing a worm. Every time you catch a fish, you are literally deceiving it. It is as if you are saying, "Come on my friend, I will feed you!" But when it comes to you, you hook and kill it. Can you say that it is a love offering? The animals we kill hate us. If our food brings hatred, we cannot develop love." - Sri Swami Satchidananda

Actually, just recently I stumbled upon an online newspaper article[8] about an abattoir worker who in claiming not to be able to afford veterinary costs, cut the throat of his own puppy. The result? Five months in prison! And to think, with society's blessing, he'd made his living from slaughtering!

Many of us have had the experience of admiring a field full of sheep and new born lambs. They are so undeniably cute and full of fluffiness, with such apparent, eager zest for life. We point them out to our children, joyfully observing their frolicsome glee, and then go home and eat bits of one.

Chopped!

And yet, rarely, barely, is any of this ever even given a second thought.

> Mary had a little Lamb,
> she also had tomatoes,
> she covered them in greasy sauce,
> and fried them with potatoes.

Some pranksters in Brazil set up a mock stall in a supermarket, selling freshly made sausages. They offered free, taste testing samples, and then had a machine that would churn out freshly made sausages to sell. As the machine emptied, they would pick up a live baby pig, place her in the machine, and continue churning out fresh pork sausage. Of course, the piglets weren't really being transformed on the fly to sausage, but customers were ignorant of this. Consumer reaction was one of typical cognitive dissonance. Confusion, shock, horror, disgust, and even violence toward the butcher. Watch it for yourself here[9]. Although the video was made to get laughs, it shows the inherent state of mind of the general public, and proves that the lack of ability to understand the true issue at heart, is not one of intelligence nor knowledge, but one of denial, and refusal to empathise.

> Meat is a four legged word.

I think the Indian born British comedian, playwright and vegetarian, Spike Milligan summed it up pretty well when toying with a poem by William Blake, he penned these four short lines of verse:

> *If a robin redbreast in a cage*
> *Puts all heaven in a rage*
> *How feels heaven when*
> *Dies the millionth battery hen?*

Confronted with these incontestably paradoxical attitudes toward our animal brethren, people come up with all manner of illogical reasons to justify human behaviour. For instance, some might attempt to justify things by explaining that animals, unlike humans, are basically instinctive creatures. Thus, if we find ourselves empathising unduly with them, we are guilty of anthropomorphising; giving them qualities which are clearly unique to us intellectually superior humans.

The truth is, there is nought wrong with anthropomorphising. Indeed, other species have much more in common with humans than we regularly care to admit. Anthropomorphising rightly leads to

27

developing more empathy toward members of other species.

Every pet owner can vouch for this. They know that each animal is endowed with his own peculiarities. They know that when a pet

> Teach a man to fish and you teach him to kill.

looks sad, bored or hurt, he is probably indeed sad, bored or hurt. There is no rocket science in this. These are far from being uniquely human attributes and are shared with pretty much every animal out there, regardless of species. One no more has the right to deny such emotions in other species than a solipsist has the right to deny the emotions of other humans. The fact that animals cannot say "I am hurt" (in any human language) does not mean they do not hurt.

The dark-aged, primitive society we live in, loves to push the theory that we need to eat flesh. As much as the industry that produces it may perhaps be a little gory for some, many choose to view it as a necessary and unavoidable fact of life. In seriously challenging this supposed fact, those who propose it are at a loss to adequately defend their stance. Nutritionally, their argument mostly revolves loosely around protein and vitamin B12.

As stated in the Introduction, my preference is not to get involved with a nutritional science that I personally find untrustworthy, but rather I intend to stick with simplicity and ethics. A certain percentage of this world live their lives never really partaking in flesh. Estimates vary as to what percentage of the world is

> "Sometimes people hold a core belief that is very strong. When they are presented with evidence that works against the belief, the new evidence cannot be accepted. It would create a feeling that is extremely uncomfortable, called cognitive dissonance. And because it is important to protect the core belief, they will rationalize, ignore and even deny anything that doesn't fit in with the core belief." - Frantz Fanon

vegetarian, but there seems to be a generally accepted agreement that the figure lies somewhere between five and ten percent of the world's population. Their life expectancy, by some estimates is reportedly higher than that of the average omnivore[10]. Personally, I have no need to seek further evidence. I understand that people can live at least lives of average lengths (or longer), even more healthily, without ever adopting zombie-like flesh eating habits. Therefore I have no issue in dismissing any claims that one must eat flesh.

In the newly revised Australian Dietary Guidelines released this year (2013), Australia's top health experts now agree with leading health advisory boards in the US and Canada, that well-planned vegan diets are a safe, healthy and viable option for all age groups.[11]

Another commonly-voiced supposed reason as to why it's acceptable to eat animals, is that they blatantly exist to be eaten, as this is just *nature's way*. Bears eat fish, lions eat Zebra; look around you! The world is a killing machine; there exists an undeniable food chain, and we are at the top of it. Thus we have the God-given right to eat anything beneath us.

This argument supposes that because animals eat other animals, we too should be granted the same privileges. Logically this implies that being indifferent to human suffering should also be acceptable behaviour; a crocodile wouldn't help a drowning human, why should we? Other animals do lots of things we might consider immoral. There is no jungle law prohibiting any behaviour, regardless of how gross we deem it to be. Murder, rape, theft, incest etc; it all happens. So should we argue that everything which happens in nature be allowed within human society? While we are looking up to animals as model citizens to mimic, should we eat our own faeces too, like dogs sometimes do? And while, obviously, many animals are natural born carnivores and omnivores, comparative anatomy indicates that we are physiologically herbivore/frugivore[12].

> "The animals of the world exist for their own reasons. They were not made for humans any more than black people were made for white, or women were created for men." - Alice Walker

I say forget the folly of looking up to other species as examples as to how we should or shouldn't behave. Instead we need to begin to think for ourselves, and there is no more meaningful philosophy than to treat others as we ourselves would ultimately prefer to be treated.

Ask yourself, would it be okay for someone to imprison you, fatten you up by feeding you crap and then ultimately slaughter and butcher you for supper? Of course not! I would not be happy with this and neither would you, nor anyone else. Now ask yourself why you might find it tolerable for other individuals of other species to endure such treatment and untimely death? Seriously ask yourself, because without empathy, there can be no compassion!

If you answer that animals do not share the awareness and intelligence of humans, then surely by this logic small children, the mentally retarded and comatose people also do not deserve rights to protection,

29

since they also can neither reason nor formulate ethical positions as mentally healthy adult humans are able.

Don't be mistaken and believe I am talking now purely of death and dying. This inevitable fate awaits us all. I am talking strictly about immoral imprisonment of innocent sentience[13] and their final cold blooded murder.

> "Anyone who says he can see through women is missing a lot."
> - Groucho Marx

Speciesism

I am not the first to propose this, but the only genuine reason I can see that such behaviour toward other species is sanctioned, is that the bulk of humankind are speciesists. Similar to the chauvinists, whose belief is that the opposite gender is basically inferior, the ageists who discriminate others because of their age and the racists whose belief is that certain races, or those of a certain skin tone are inherently inferior, the speciesists believe it is perfectly normal and just to abuse other beings purely because they are not human. There is, of course, no logic, no rational reasoning, behind drawing such conclusions. There is no logic in deciding what's acceptable and permissible in disregarding the needs of certain selected animal species.

In practice, within the western world at least, there are really only a few predominant species which are singled out and subjected to lives of torment; cows, pigs, sheep, chicken and a couple of handfuls of aquatic

> How many would protest if restaurants began serving puppy and kitten flesh instead of calves? Robins instead of hens? Squirrels instead of pigs?

species probably receive the bulk of the abuse. If factory farming for meat of cats, dogs, squirrels, swans and guinea pigs[14] began in western Europe, you can be sure some of the bacon and sausage gorging public would be out protesting. Although other cultures regularly eat some or all of these animals, everybody draws the line somewhere. Most would balk at the idea of eating dolphin, gorilla, orangutan or human flesh, but really the differences between the species are minimal and whether we are a rabbit, horse, chimpanzee or human, we all have an innate desire to live our lives freely and avoid violation.

I say put aside backgrounds, traditions and cultures, because they are often unexplored reasons behind the discriminatory choices made.

Instead, empathise with your victim, and put yourself in her or his place. Would you be content if nobody did anything to deliver you from such a life of evil and torment?

Faced With The Facts

By being forced to truly confront the cold hard

> Look a pig in his eyes, and understand the truth behind bacon.

facts behind meat production[15], I strongly believe that the majority of people, especially in the western world, would cringe and feel disgust, likely also shame.

I think this world would stand to benefit from sending everyone on a slaughterhouse visit at least once in their life. Or at least if we could all take time out to watch Gary Yourofsky's inspirational speech on youtube[16] or EARTHLINGS[17]. I don't mean to just watch the first three minutes, walk away in disgust and try to put it behind us, but to actually watch it from beginning to end and ponder deeply over the role all of us have unwittingly played in it through sponsoring such action via the goods we have bought as unwitting consumers. Of course, the ultimate vision is that there should be no such thing as a slaughterhouse, or an EARTHLINGS video, but until that day comes, it would bode us well to witness the reality and to reflect deeply upon it.

> "Freethinkers are those who are willing to use their minds without prejudice and without fearing to understand things that clash with their own customs, privileges, or beliefs. This state of mind is not common, but it is essential for right thinking; Where it is absent, discussion is apt to become worse than useless." - Leo Tolstoy

Tolstoy Story

I am reminded of a little story I once read somewhere about Tolstoy, the Russian author of *War and Peace*, a renowned vegetarian of his era.

Apparently, his aunt once complained consistently throughout a meal he had prepared for her, due to the blatant absence of any meat to sink her teeth into.

Tolstoy, a man of many thoughts, pondered over this dilemma and on a subsequent occasion of cooking for her, she was pleasantly surprised to be informed that she would be served chicken.

His aunt, no doubt gleefully anticipating her meal, arrived at the table only to find a live chicken tied to the leg of her chair, and a butcher's knife waiting on the table. Tolstoy answered her fluster by stating: "All you have to do is slaughter the animal, and we will be glad to prepare her for you."

The story goes, that being also vegetarian by nature, though clearly ignorant of the fact, the aunt was unable to end the chicken's life, and from that point on, ceased eating meat.[18]

Thought Experiment

> By eating the flesh of another, we are effectively turning our body into the grave of another. - R.I.P.

Test yourself. Picture this. You are hungry and before you is a live chicken and a very sharp knife. Are you capable/willing to take the life of the chicken yourself? If yes, could you truly do so without riddling your conscience with guilt, or, later or immediate, feelings of sadness, regret or remorse?

I'm not too naïve to realise that there are some people out there, that would stand up and answer yes, that they could do so, even gladly, but what I adamantly refuse to believe is that they would be being totally honest with themselves about not feeling the slightest sentiment of regret.

Avoid muddying the issue and don't think of it as a do or die situation! Imagine you have a fridge full of vegan food.

> "The idea that some lives matter less, is the root of all that is wrong with the world" - Dr. Paul Farmer

Flesh Eating is a Cowardly Practice

In my opinion, Flesh-Eating is generally a cowardly practice. I say this, because, like Tolstoy's aunt, few of us are genuinely prepared to personally confront the stone cold bloodiness of murder.

We get others to do the work that we ourselves are unable to do, because in our hearts we all know how ignoble an act it is, to deprive another of his life. Even the slaughterhouse workers are not ignorant of the ignobility of murder. Witnessing endless carnage day after mind-numbing day is utterly devastating to one's mental well-being, frequently resulting in post-traumatic stress disorder. Such a "job" will inevitably drain one's physical, emotional, mental and spiritual well-being. To be constantly surrounded by the animals' heart wrenching cries for help as well as their blood, urine and faeces, cannot *not* pay its toll. Desensitisation is pretty inevitable for anyone that can take the job over a longer period and purportedly also results in unprovoked episodes of rage and anger. (directed toward other humans too)[19].

There is a reason we shield our children from the murderous facts behind their meals. We know that they still know, they have yet to be corrupted and should they be faced with the truth, will recognise the disturbing blood-lust of life taking[20]. They have yet to be desensitised.

I recall a young girl I used to babysit back in the 1980s. She once witnessed her father remove a transparent plastic bag from the freezer. Its contents were a mangled portion of a lamb's carcass. After a while, as the bone and flesh began to thaw, blood settled at the bottom of the bag. Three year old Claire looked at it and said in all innocence: "Is that lamb's juice?". Her father looked at her and calmly answered: "No my love, that's lamb's blood". Claire was silent for a brief moment, then with all conviction, replied "I don't want to ever eat that again.". Of course, within a week her father had rationally and patiently convinced his daughter that it was *perfectly normal* and quite necessary to eat meat, and thus had helped her on her path of increasing desensitisation.

While our inner temperaments may be truly Divine, our souls are constantly in a state of tumultuous unrest due to the atrocities our lifestyles help support and perpetuate.

Golden Buddha

I'm reminded of another apparently true story I heard once. It transpired some decades ago in Bangkok, Thailand.

> Old MacDonald had a farm.
> Yowie, Owie, Ow!...
> With some bloody flesh here,
> And a squawk squawk there,
> Hear a squeal. Hear a screech.
> Everywhere a death zone.

The government had decided to build a major road through a certain area of the city. Unfortunately it just so happened that a pre-eminent Buddhist monastery stood right in the path of the proposed highway. A relocation was thus in order. Now, it also happened that within the walls of this monastery, there stood a giant clay statue of a rounded Buddha also requiring relocation.

Initial attempts to lift the statue with a crane resulted in cracks appearing on the side of the Buddha. Not desiring to damage the statue further, the attempt was abandoned as they paused to reconsider their options. That night, it began to rain and fearing the rain would widen the crack, one monk set about covering the statue. During his efforts to protect the effigy, he suddenly notice something glittering from within the crack. Curiosity getting the better of him, he cautiously widened the crack to discover gold. Widening the crack yet further, he realised that the whole statue was solid gold with just a surface layer of clay.

Historians supposed that at some point in time, monks had covered the statue in clay to hide it from invading foreign forces and that they themselves likely all fell victim to those forces, thus the secret of the Buddha was lost until the fateful day, centuries later, when the government decided their city needed a bypass.

This is how I picture us all to be. Born into the dementia of this asylum, the inner golden purity of our souls becomes gradually and increasingly more encrusted by negativity and dirt, until our shining true qualities are so suppressed and forgotten that we can no longer even recognise ourselves. If only a simple intercity bypass would suffice to make us realise the truth!

Hidden Industry

Shortly before starting on the writing of this book, while exercising my innate nomadic nature, I journeyed through South-east Asia. There, I witnessed skinned cats and dogs hanging from

"As with any violent ideology, the populace must be shielded from direct exposure to the victims of the system, lest they begin questioning the system or their participation in it. This truth speaks for itself: Why else should the meat industry go to such lengths to keep its practices invisible?" - Melanie Joy

hooks and stall after stall of dying and dead fish, eels and chickens etc. Their carcasses fly infested and rotting in the tropical heat. People carrying chickens tied together, hanging upside down by their feet, *still alive*, but only barely. Sights that have long passed from being common place within the traditional western market.

It dawned on me just how much the animal exploitation industries in the west have become increasingly more concealed.

I believe this increasingly gradual concealment has been a natural consequence of the equally increasing rise in empathy and vegetarianism throughout the western world and has been, in essence, a necessity for the animal abusers, as they are fully aware that should the grizzly facts become open and publicly visible, ever more people would choose not to eat the flesh of other beings.

Thus the more sensitive the masses become, the more the meat industry is forced to hide its bloody goriness. Choosing instead tactics like cleverly presenting their wares on neutral, neatly packaged, sterile polystyrene trays, wrapped in clear plastic.

Even the words we use to describe the flesh we eat veils the frank bloody facts, instead of eating cows, we eat beef. Instead of eating calves, we eat veal, instead of eating pigs, we eat ham, pork and bacon, instead of sheep, we eat mutton. Curiously enough, etymologically, many of these words come from the French words for the animals themselves: veau/calf/veal, boeuf/ox/bullock/beef, mouton/sheep/mutton, porc/pig/swine/pork

Then there are those who in futile attempts to appease vegetarian thoughts, console themselves with the notion that should an animal be murdered in the right way, with the right ritual performed and a prayer said afterwards, that the animal will actually benefit from being slaughtered as the animal's soul will be given the opportunity to rise to planes hitherto unobtainable for him.

> "Saying "eating animals is yummy" as a justification for killing them, is pretty much the same as saying rape is okay since it feels good to the rapist. Civilized people require more than sensory pleasure to justify behaviours." - Stephanie Theisen

Beside the fact that I've yet to actually meet someone who, with all knowledge and forethought, genuinely consistently seeks out such slaughtered flesh, in my eyes this is nought more than another clever ploy to dampen the growing concern amidst the all too gullible masses.

There is no Right Way to Murder Anyone

Look at it this way, if I invite you around to live at our place, let you eat freely from our trees, clothe you and give you comfort and companionship for several years, and then one day call you inside and shoot you, butcher you up and eat your rump with scrambled eggs, would it suddenly make everything hunky-dory if I went around saying, "It's okay you know, I fully respected the dude, I treated him well, he had a good time here. Shucks, I even listened to him while he talked of his philosophy on

> "When I despair, I remember that all through history the way of truth and love have always won. There have been tyrants and murderers, and for a time, they can seem invincible, but in the end, they always fall. Think of it; always." - Mahatma Gandhi

life and showed me his boring vacation photos, and don't forget he ate whatever fruit he wanted from my trees. I even blessed his body after slaughtering him *and* said a little prayer so his spirit could move on to higher plains! Rest assured, I killed him with love!"

Let's face the facts squarely and not try to hide behind some notion of ceremony or ritual, the reason I invited you around was never out of respect for you, it was to fatten you up and shank you. When I saw you, it was not as a friend or an equal, or even as another being, it was as part of a devilishly greasy three course meal, and when I made sure the wicked wolf didn't get you, it was only so I could do so instead.

One conclusion that can be drawn from traditional tribal ritual performed upon or after the killing of an animal, is that those participating recognise that the act of taking another's life is not something taken lightly and there is acknowledgement that something is not right with it.

> "Awareness is bad for the meat business. Conscience is bad for the meat business. Sensitivity to life is bad for the meat business. DENIAL, however, the meat business finds indispensable" - John Robbins

No matter how you look at it though, murder is murder and regardless of what prayers are said, murder is always committed without the consent of the victim. Hiding behind the unshakeably unknowable destiny of another's soul is a poor excuse at the best of times, and would likely not appease your own theoretical untimely assassination even if someone were to assure you that your soul would benefit from taking a shot to the head. Stop kidding yourself!

> "You must be the change you wish to see in the world" - Mahatma Gandhi

Slavery

Bear the following in mind again:

Barely a century and a half ago, it was considered a reasonable practice by many in the west and elsewhere, to forcibly capture people from certain regions of the globe and to thereafter freight them elsewhere, whereby they would sold and beaten into accepting their fates as slaves.

People were, as the saying goes, treated like animals. But let's face it, not even animals deserve to be "treated like animals", in this fashion. Now a hundred and fifty years further down the track, if we look back at those happenings at all, we probably do so with bafflement and grief, that our ancestors could so easily have gone about their daily affairs, discussing the weather, while other people not too far down the road, were being beaten and tortured into accepting lifetimes completely not of their own choosing. Meanwhile still, yet other fore-parents, were actually trading in stocks of freighted people. Fine young specimens!

Who among us is able to put their hand up and say they honestly believe, that what we were doing back then was right and just, and would be happy to rekindle those old habits? Sure, there may well be a few die hard triple K members still floating around out there that regret that the trade ever lost legal status[a], but these shouldn't seriously be considered good role models for the masses. Besides, although mostly illegal, a multibillion-dollar slave industry is still very much in existence today. In fact there are said to be more people enslaved now than ever before in history[21].

It is one of my profound beliefs, that there will come a day, hopefully not too far off, when we will all look back at the relationship we currently have with animals, and be sick to our teeth about how we have used and treated them. Or, more appropriately, abused and mistreated them.

> (on fish) "Now I can look at you in peace; I don't eat you any more." - Franz Kafka

How we have deprived them of their freedoms, their natural environments, their families. How we have fed them grossly unnatural diets, regularly restricted their movements to tiny booths, stalls and cages, where they have been unable to even turn around. All for nothing less than the sake of gluttony, hearing aids and heart attacks; side dishes to our cheese and ham sandwiches (if that makes no sense to you now, as I'm aware I'm getting a little ahead of myself here, then hopefully it will become clearer as you read on through the pages of this book).

> Two goldfish are in a tank. One turns to the other and says, "Do you know how to drive this thing?"

In Defence of the Fish

I have met many people who have taken first steps toward vegetarianism but continue the struggle to justify feasting on fish flesh.

There is no doubt in my mind that fish too are individuals, struggling to stay alive and unharmed, with as much aversion toward pain and captivity as any other animal species.

What a horror it must be to be caught up and cramped in nets, and forced to slowly suffocate in the air, or feel that yanking realisation that the morsel of food we just ate has an embedded hook within it.

---

a   The slave industry is still very much in existence. In fact, there are said to be more people enslaved now than ever before in history. The difference between then and now, however, is that the current slave trade is vastly invisible and all takes place without the consent of current, global, legal systems.

A Fishy Story

Imagine you are of a slightly different intelligence, walking along some street, happily anticipating lunch and just generally minding your own business, when suddenly you come across a slice of pizza, seemingly suspended in mid-air by some unseen force.

> "I know the human being and fish can co-exist peacefully."
> - George W. Bush (I have no idea where he was going with that one, but surely he is right!)

You sniff the pizza and your demented sense of smell tells you it smells good. You take a bite. Yeah. Good stuff! Soon you've devoured the whole slice and wondering where the next one will appear from.

But there is an annoying hair on your tongue. You try to pull at it and suddenly there is a sharp pain from deep within your throat. This is shortly followed by an additional unexpected "tug", and the next thing you know, you cough up a mouthful of blood and your body is yanked irresistibly upward.

> What's the difference between a fish and a guitar? You can't tuna fish.

Meanwhile, up on the eighth floor of the block beside you, some geezer, cigarette dripping from his lips, baseball cap on backwards, leaning back on his stool, is reading his newspaper. He sees a movement on his line. Folds up his newspaper, tucks it under the one leg of his stool and starts reeling in.

Horrific what? I suppose you can be quite sure that the average cod with the average chips, has not been caught in this fashion, but more likely has been trapped by a net and pulled out of the water with thousands or more of her brethren and left to steadily suffocate. Flapping around spasmodically, slowly and painfully asphyxiating.

> "Everybody is a genius. But if you judge a fish by its ability to climb a tree, it will live its whole life believing that it's stupid." - Albert Einstein

Either way you look at it, not too nice a scene. But let's face it, truthful. Those that call Fishing a "sport", have to realise that there is nothing remotely "cricket" about it.

Yes, kid yourself no longer that you need to eat animals to live! This is an absurd notion. This is what is meant by the expression, *believe absurdities and you will commit atrocities*. It does not have to be this way!

Carnage Statistics

Human lust for flesh based foods causes the murder of literally tens of billions of animals annually. Roughly sixty billion land based animals alone are killed yearly. Factor in also water living creatures, and the figure soars to over hundred billion! That's a shocking 100,000,000,000 animals whose lives are cut short purely for human gluttony[22]. The US alone is responsible for more than ten percent of that number, with twenty three million chickens and one hundred thousand cows (over four thousand every hour) killed daily[23]! These figures are surely a conservative estimation, and by some reckoning, the massacre toll is said to be even higher. This website[24] for example, states that in 2011, including shellfish, sixty three billion animals lost their lives to feed Americans alone. And see here[25] for a very disturbing real time counter of globally slain animals. The truly accurate kill statistics are beyond counting, but to be sure, the majority of victims suffer far more intensely than most homicide victims, these are murders you'll not find mentioned in the daily tabloids. It's time for us all to face up to these facts and acknowledge the unwitting role we've all played in shaping them.

> Most people just want to be left in peace to eat their bacon, not realising that there is no *peace* behind bacon.

Flesh Alternatives

If you are perchance currently a shod omnivore, and I've somehow managed to reach your better sensibilities, leaving you with desire to take this first step on the path to Eden, but desperately craving steak like food, then be aware the market is flooded with alternatives to ease one over to the vegetarian diet. Many are bean based, and can be prepared and eaten in much the same way as animal derived sinews and thews, you can even buy rashes of soy bacon and mince-meat-similar TVP (Textured Vegetable Protein). Scientists (bless their precious cotton socks!), have now succeeded in fully synthesising meat in a laboratory[26]. And the very latest news, hot off the presses, is that bioprinters may soon be able to print meat[27]! There is NO valid reason to continue supporting the flesh trade.

Why choose to harm, when there are
other things to eat, drink and wear?

VEGANISM

Now, although becoming vegetarian is surely a good step toward bringing more peace to this planet, as an ethical dietary choice, it is somewhat lacking and rather hypocritical. Hence veganism steps in to iron out the flaws and crinkles of vegetarianism.

> "The standard diet of a meat-eater is blood, flesh, veins, muscles, tendons, cow secretions, hen periods and bee vomit. And once a year during a certain holiday in November, meat-eaters use the hollowed-out rectum of a dead bird as a pressure cooker for stuffing. And people think vegans are weird because we eat tofu?" - Gary Yourofsky

Defining Veganism

I've been wanting to write this for some time now. I want to make it very clear from the onset, that veganism, despite frequent claims contrarily, is not and never has been, a diet.

So, you know how some people say that they are vegan for health reasons? Or vegan for environmental reasons? Or even vegan for social reasons?

Well, technically speaking, they're all wrong!

Wrong, that is, unless they have redefined the term veganism from that which it was originally intended. Which of course, is what has colloquially happened to many words becoming misused and abused as is the plight of the daily spoken English language. So, on second thoughts, perhaps that makes them right in a sense[28]. But not if one takes the literal meaning of the word as it was first coined back in the 1940s.

I believe the original definition went something like this:

VEGANISM may be defined as a way of living which seeks to exclude, as far as possible and practical, all forms of exploitation of, and cruelty to, animals for food, clothing or any other purpose[29].

> "It's troubling when people get upset with vegans for pointing out the suffering, rather than getting upset with themselves for causing it." - Jo Tyler

Yes, I admit, if you followed the last link, you'll have noticed that I deliberately left out the part of how, in dietary terms veganism is generally further defined as the practice of dispensing with all animal produce, including meat, fish, poultry, eggs, animal milks, honey and their derivatives, but only because the real golden rule is to leave animals be! As a moral philosophy though, I would say that veganism has no clear definitive rule forbidding even the eating of animal flesh! I see no fundamental moral rule that would prevent, for example, the eating of an accidental road-kill!

Veganism is a lifestyle choice that attempts to minimise undue suffering toward animals!

Real Men Don't Eat Quiche

> "My body will not be a tomb for other creatures." - Leonardo Da Vinci

When you think about it, vegetarianism, or veg"eat-dairy"anism as one friend once so wittily put it, is a very human diet; at least as it is put in to practice by the majority of adherents out there.

(Note: that was *human* diet, not to be confused with *humane*).

What I mean by this, is that no other animal species consciously chooses to not eat the flesh of another, but still imprisons winged beings to systematically steal their eggs to fry, ending their lives prematurely after egg yield begins to diminish, and does likewise with large mammals, raising them until child bearing age, systematically raping them and forcefully separating mother and child in order to carton off the milk, rightfully intended for the offspring and send it to the waiting dairy crazed milky masses. - White and two sugars?

And further, the human animal will happily go out and buy the flayed skin of a slaughtered innocent, skilfully fashioned into footwear, trousers, skirts, belts, jackets, gloves and handbags.

Again, I'd like to clearly underline that the true essence of veganism is not about diet, and thus offers no clear guidelines as to how the diet of a follower should or shouldn't be.

> "People eat meat and think they will become as strong as an ox, forgetting that the ox eats grass." - Pino Caruso

There is no underlying concern if the diet is raw or cooked, condimented or plain, mixed or mono, toxic or palatable, rotten, ripe or unripe, deep fried, roasted, boiled, sautéed, smoked, alcohol fortified, preserved, MSG flavour enhanced, coloured, fermented, pasteurised, curried, sugared, spiced or just plain natural. Provided of course, no animal was exploited during its production!

Of course, referring to the road kill example I just gave, finding and eating dead animals on the side of the road is not something any vegan I've ever know was in to. I would imagine that most would find the same kind of repulsiveness to the proposition as they would when faced with eating their own naturally dead grandmother.

My point is that veganism per sé, has little outlying regard or concern for the health of those that practise it. Don't get me wrong, I am not saying that vegans aren't concerned for their own health, of course they are, who really isn't? Who doesn't want to live a long, prosperous and contented healthy life?

All I am saying is that those claiming to be vegan for health reasons, do so not for concerns stemming from the philosophy of veganism or any of its original guidelines, but from their own will to live happily and healthily.

Actually, the English language is really missing a word to describe someone that purely eats a diet free of animal products. The French for example, in addition to the word veganisme, have the word vegetalisme, which describes the philosophy of just eating solely from the vegetable kingdom. So they have vegetarisme, vegetalisme and veganisme. Similarly, the Spaniards do the same, with the words vegetarismo, vegetalismo and veganismo. I guess the English equivalent of vegetalismo would have to be dietary veganism.

So, put simply, veganism is an attempt to avoid being the cause of unnecessary animal suffering.

> "Excellence is never an accident. It is always the result of high intention, sincere effort, and intelligent execution; it represents the wise choice of many alternatives - choice, not chance, determines your destiny." - Aristotle

Dairy Cows

I've met so many vegetarians, some of them extremely sensitive individuals who knew instinctively from very young ages that eating the flesh from someone else's body, just wasn't cricket.

Surprisingly though, many of them are very reluctant to hear the truth about dairy. In their hearts, they must see that something is wrong with it, but their stomachs really don't want to listen. They conveniently prefer to remain totally ignorant of the facts. Cheese, yoghurt and eggs are, in many ways, just as addictive and harmful as, or perhaps even more so, than flesh products.

Actually, it is my firm belief that in reality production of these items may be causing more cruelty and suffering to our fellow brethren than does the trade in their flesh. It may, for example, be argued, that flesh can conceivably be gotten from bodies whose original owners have lived freely in their natural habitats until one fateful day when a bullet retires them early.

On the other hand, the same can never be said of milk products. Please don't be mislead to believe otherwise. The milk-for-human's animals' shelf life lasts only while the being is able to produce large enough quantities of milk to satisfy the financial desires of the producers. Naturally this is only until the biological end of the animal's peak offspring rearing years. For cows this means being forced pregnant from as early an age as possible, each year, for roughly 5 years, at which point they are deemed no longer ideal and thus slaughtered.

> 50% of all chickens hatched and calves born are male. What do you believe is the fate of the vast majority of those males? Why do you think it's so rare to see fields full of bulls, or cages packed full of roosters? http://bit.ly/ChickBelt and http://bit.ly/DairyFacts

No other animal species takes milk naturally after leaving the stage of dependency on the mother.

Yet, somehow, the mass marketing, advertising industry has completely hoodwinked the majority of us, into believing we need milk all our lives and that should we miss out, we will undoubtedly suffer from the lack of it.

Still Breast Feeding at Ten Years Old

Hmmpf! Examine your feelings when you hear about the hypothetical woman still breastfeeding her own child at ten years old. Now go and open your fridge door! Are you telling vegans to grow up and get a life? Open your fridge door! Grow up and wean yourself!

The molecular constituency of cow's milk is so radically different to that of a human mother's milk, that calves quadruple their weight within the first months of their lives. Ponder over the origins of childhood obesity!

Cows are pumped full of hormones and antibiotics in order to increase milk yield and stop infections, mastitis etc. Many of these chemicals are transferred via the host into the milk. Milk after weaning[30] is a highly unnatural food for us and any other animal species, milk from another species, even more so, and pasteurised hormone saturated milk from another species even further so.

43

The average modern dairy cow regularly produces between thirty five to fifty litres a day[31]. Even one cow recently is reported to be producing a staggering one hundred litres of milk a day[32]. Udders dragging back-cripplingly heavily on dirty floors.

> Milk comes from a grieving mother.

Chickens

Natural chickens running wild in their native non interfered settings have been observed to produce an average of six to twelve eggs every few months, all of which, generally speaking, hatch into fluffy young chicks.

Contrarily, chickens in farms however, have been known to lay in excess of three hundred eggs a year! A feat that cannot possibly *not* have a toll on the mother's poor enslaved body.

A single battery farm can contain hundreds of thousands of battery hens, stacked in cages five rows high in enclosed sheds. These hens suffer intensely and continuously throughout their short miserable lives. A battery hen may spend her entire life, laying cramped inside a shared cage, each containing three to twenty hens. Each hen's floor area is equivalent to little more than one A4 sheet of paper[33]. With her wings outstretched, a hen is twice the size of a typical battery cage. Read more here[34].

> If you love the creator, take care of her creatures/creations

Knowing these facts, some people might choose to eat free range or organic chickens and eggs, believing them to be given a fair deal. Sadly they are misinformed. To increase profits, many free-range (and organic!) farms cram literally thousands of their chickens on mud-filled lots or together in sheds with a simple access door to the outside, that only the closest chickens get to use[35]. These animals often suffer through the same mutilations, (debeaking) without painkillers, that occur on factory farms. Actually by some accounts, due to the extreme overcrowding and filthy conditions, organically raised chickens sometimes suffer from higher mortality rates than their drugged battery farmed equivalents and due to the lack of antibiotics, can end up with even more parasites than are found in factory chickens.

Each one of those chickens has her own thoughts, her own unique personality and individuality, experiencing little more than endless discomfort and merciless unremitting agony..

Leather and Cheese

The hide of cows can sometimes make up ten percent of the animal's gross financial value. Kid yourself no longer that leather is just a side product of the industry[36]. It is as much part and parcel of the animal's ultimate suffering, as is the trade in her flesh and the grinding of her bones for gelatin.

Due to the rennet ingredient, taken from the stomach of the slaughtered animal (often from the slaughtered young), the vast majorities of cheeses should not even be considered vegetarian.

Wool and Silk

I think it's pretty obvious how fur farms work[37] so see no reason to write more on that. But one animal covering which is often little understood is wool[38]. Many may erroneously believe that it's gotten without harm to the sheep, but the wool industry too is yet another demonstration of animal exploitation. The sheep (and in some cases goats and rabbits [39]) are bred and valued for one main purpose; their wool. When the wool diminishes, they too are sent on a one way trip to a slaughterhouse. To my knowledge, shearers are never paid by the hour, but by the number of sheep they shear, thus the incentive is to get through each sheep as quickly as possible, very rough handling. There are more issues to be aware of too. Read more here.[40]

Silk worms are bred and killed by the hundreds of millions yearly. Thrown into boiling water, roughly fifteen are needed to produce just one gram of silk[41]!

The Best Kept Cows

"All beings tremble before violence. All fear death, all love life. See yourself in others. Then whom can you hurt? What harm can you do." - Buddha

To make clearer the plight of even the best kept cows, I'd like to tell you the following short story. Although told from the view point of a cow (I might add one of the luckier ones who avoided the factory farm), it is actually a very true

45

story, based on actual occurrences. The one man in the story referred to as the Gentle One is completely non-fictional and it is through his recounting of events that I penned this story.

My Life as a Cow

Spring had once more descended upon us and for the second time during my brief existence, I found myself heavy with child.

Birds chorused their spring melodies and the wind bore its sweet, fresh fragrance. The only evidence remaining of the cold winter passed, were the odd patches of snow framed by silver linings of melting ice at which the sun slowly etched.

We had seen none of it though. Winter has been a season we were never given the chance to know. Imprisoned indoors, confined to small booths. But with the commencement of spring, we were once more ushered outside to the waiting grass, sun and above all, renewed hope.

Within me, I felt my child's restricted movements. Its ever increasing impatience, gently but forcefully informing me that birth was imminent. With encouragement, I sent out feelings of love, to wait, to be patient. Not yet, the time was not quite right.

> Rather than grate cheese, we should belittle it!

My thoughts, without words, but thoughts none-the-less, retreated to the events of the previous year. Spring had barely begun and after just a very fleeting moment of contact, my first born had been forcibly separated from me. Who knows what fate awaited her. I mourned the loss for many weeks, searching for her, calling desperately. But to no avail, never did I see her again.

But they were happenings of the year past and although I still remembered (indeed, how could I possibly have forgotten?), time had slowly healed over the wounds of this traumatic loss. Make no doubts, this is a hard and cruel life I have lead. Only the simple pleasures

> Just beautiful!
> His mother sighed,
> The day that he was born;
> His velvet eyes, his curly hair,
> his darling baby form
> **************
> Just beautiful! Another cried.
> (That very same sweet babe).
> She licked her greasy lips,
> then washed him down
> with lemonade.

have kept me sane throughout it all. I did not suffer alone. My sisters offered warmth and gentleness, though their circumstances were clearly no better than my own. They too have suffered the loss of their children at the merciless hands of humans. But I would not give up hope. I could not.

During the autumn, before the air turned cold and we were moved permanently indoors, the new one arrived. The Gentle-one. Unlike the Rough-handed-one, his voice did not bellow, showed signs of kindness and contained reassuring words of comfort. He would visit us daily, offering soft words and firm neck-strokes. He attached the plastic tubes to the teats of my udder with more care and consideration. Though truthfully the milking was always more of a frustrating cold ordeal never a pleasing experience and I was always glad when this was over. Please don't underestimate my intelligence, I know what I have missed and for who my milk was truly intended.

Yes, I held hope that the Gentle-one could help. I believed he would understand and as the time drew close, I silently left my sisters and headed toward the stream where I could see him working in a neighbouring field.

"Mmoo"

"Oh, it's you Emily, you gave me a fright. What are you doing down here. you know you should be in the other field with the rest of the herd. Come along now, get back with you."

Of course, his words meant little to me, but his intention

"I spent 45 years in the cattle industry, always professing that I loved my animals. But it was years before I was willing to admit that I was more interested in profit than the animals' health. The fact of it is, we simply raised them to a point where they became economically beneficial for us to sell. I finally woke up. Looking in those big old brown eyes, I realised that those animals loved life in their own way, just as I loved life in mine. There was no way in the world I could ever put them to death again" - Howard Lyman

was clear, he wanted me to return. He pushed my head gently backwards and slapped my side firmly, encouraging me to leave. However, his voice seemed neither harsh, nor reprimanding, so I stood my ground firmly, aware that the birth was only minutes away.

"Come along now Ems, don't be a silly girl, I don't have all day, there's work to be done here, can't you see. Best you be getting back now."

More friendly words and gentle attempts at persuasion but he didn't seem to mind my presence too much, so I stood firm and waited.

"Okay, stay there if you wish, but don't come too close, or you'll be liable to hurt yourself"

He turned once more to his work and whistled contentedly and, I believed, soon forgot about my presence. After a while, I felt movement within me. Very quickly and smoothly, my son entered the world. Bloody and small and helpless. I licked his face clearing a passage for air to enter his nostrils and mouth and cleaned around his eyes and ears. My son, no one could deny the love bond between us. I smelt him, cleaned him, loved him and as our bodies moved closer, he found my udder and took his first taste of its rich milk. This is what I had been missing, this gentle creatures tongue at my udder. I let out a "Mooo" of ecstasy.

"Yes, hallo Emily. Well, what have we here? A mighty fine looking young beef calf. Well done, good work Emily. He'll fetch a good price, I suppose we'd best be getting you both back"

He moved over to my son and hoisting him over his shoulders, moved off in the direction of the rest of the herd. Naturally my son was alarmed, but I mooed reassuring moos and licked him comfortingly on his neck as I followed closely beside them both. I felt quite sure that things would be different this time around.

> Think about the following:
> What do you allow yourself to eat?
> Fish? Chicken? Lamb? Pig? Dog? Donkey? Swan?
> Dolphin? Panda? Budgerigar? Chipmunk? Human?
> ---
> Quite profoundly,
> where do you draw the line?
> Why do you draw that particular line?
> Befriend an animal
> and learn its uniqueness, its individuality.
> Give a chicken a name
> and learn to love it, then strangle it yourself.
> Leg of Lamb, leg of human,
> leg of your pet cat.
> Some serious thinking may well be in order.
> **Meat Means Murder**

He put my son down and left us both standing with my sisters. three full days my second child and I spent together. On the fourth day, the two men entered the field at dawn and separated us. That afternoon, I found myself once more in a booth in the milking parlour, with tubes attached to my udder.

Severely stressed and frustrated and although the Gentle-one's voice was just as firm and soft as always, there was no more reassurance, and waves of confusion swept over me. I called out and cried for several days, often long into the night, but my cries were in vain and eventually I gave up hope of ever seeing him again. Routine life with my sisters continued and we were all able to comfort each other to an extent, as we had all suffered the same loss.

Summer arrived, and once more I found myself fastened to the rape rack. A bull, of jersey stock, brown, white and oversized, mounted me. Heavily, clumsily planting his seed within me. Though I hasten to add, I never felt, or feel, any resentment toward the bull. How could I? His lot was surely much the same as mine and my sisters. All I felt was frustrated pity.

The daily milking continued. and the touch of both humans brought forth feelings of anger and frustrated loss.

> "For to be free is not merely to cast off one's chains, but to live in a way that respects and enhances the freedom of other beings." - Nelson Mandela

Eventually, the seasons changed once more, the winds came, carrying cold air and someone saw fit to move us indoors again, keeping us locked in our small booths. Unless you have lived in one yourself for weeks/months on end, you can never understand what an experience this is. The days blend together and only the strange lighting and regular milking hours offer hints of the movement of the sun and sky outside. Those days indoors were truly the most enduring and perplexing.

For the third time in my short existence, I felt the growth of life slowly taking form within me. This only succeeded in increasing my stress. I had to be outside for the birth, to hide my child somewhere. Yes, even back then, I had the inklings of a plan forming within my mind. Naturally there was no desire to have my child stolen from me for a third time.

> "Because I'm a civil rights activist, I am also an animal rights activist. Animals and humans suffer and die alike. Violence causes the same pain, the same spilling of blood, the same stench of death, the same arrogant, cruel and vicious taking of life. We shouldn't be a part of it." - Dick Gregory

Spring arrived and we were lead outside. There was no sign of the winter having visited. No tell tale patches of snow. Perhaps the winter had been mild, or perhaps our stay indoors had been longer. We kicked our legs and breathed the clean air. So good to be outside once more. Though, as we were soon to discover, our roaming freedom had once more been restricted. An electric fence had been raised, cutting off the field to the west with the stream.

Several weeks later and the hour of birth drew nearer. Maybe tomorrow, I thought, as I sat down to sleep in the field. It was good to sleep out, to hear the wind and the insects and the gentle breathing of my sisters. Not now little one. Heavy with anticipation, I sent out feelings of love and encouragement to the child within me.

The following day, feeling the time was close and seeing a chance, I slipped away from the rest of the herd, heading for the woods. After searching around for a while, I eventually found a suitable spot. No one had seen me. I gave birth. A boy, beautiful and strong, but small and fearful. I licked his face clean and offered him my udder, but feared to stay longer lest someone should notice my absence. Alone, I returned to the field.

Later that day, the two humans came visiting.

"Looks like Em's dropped her calf, Frank"

"Yep, sure does, can't see it anywhere around though. No doubt she's hidden it somewhere. They do that on occasion. Crafty little buggers. Keep a close eye on her, no doubt she'll return to it later on."

"Sure will. Where'd you hide it eh Em? In the woods maybe? Huh? I'll go and see to the chickens, then get back to work on the tractor"

> "Being vegetarian here also means that we do not consume dairy and egg products, because they are products of the meat industry. If we stop consuming, they will stop producing. Only collective awakening can create enough determination for action." - Thich Nhat Hanh

"Okay, I'll be loading up the pigs ready for the sales this afternoon. See you later on."

I didn't know if they suspected anything or not. Perhaps they weren't even aware that I had been expecting. How was I to know how much they knew? I chewed grass with my sisters and tried to be calm.

> UN urges global move to meat and dairy-free diet. Meat and dairy products account for 70% of global freshwater consumption. 38% of the total land use and 19% of the world's greenhouse gas emissions.

Night time and darkness descended upon us and only then did I dare leave the herd and venture towards my new born son. I found him where I'd left him, sitting there, calling out to me. I nuzzled my head reassuringly against his neck. He drank thirstily from my udder, no doubt frightened and confused as to where I had been and why I had abandoned him. I licked him and moved my body closer to offer my warmth. But then, something wasn't right, movement behind me. A sister maybe? I turned around and by the light of the big round moon, saw two figures approaching through the trees.

"Here they are Pete! Knew they'd be here some place. Not the first time this has happened. Little bastard bringing us out in the middle of the night. You grab the calf and I'll get Emily back to the field."

"Mooooo"

"Okay. Looks like we got ourselves another future few hundred kilos of beef steak. Will fetch a good price at the market this one. Come along now little one, we won't hurt you."

"Mooo"

What was happening? The Gentle-one had lifted my child over his shoulders and was carrying him away from me. I

> "Compassion for animals is intimately connected with goodness of character; and it may be confidently asserted that he who is cruel to animals cannot be a good man." - Arthur Schopenhauer

tried to follow, but the Rough-handed-one barred my way and urged me roughly back in the direction of the field. My son cried out for me and in panic and confusion, I leapt forward and around, away from the rough handed one, scraping myself clumsily against branches. Eventually I worked myself free of the woods, but by then they were already halfway across the field. My son, frightened, calling out to me. Run as I might, I was unable to reach them before the gate closed. Barring my way.

I watched the Gentle-one enter the buildings with my son. I cried, I mooed, oh believe me, these were traumatic experiences. Have you ever had your child removed from you and not been able to do a thing about it? My experience was none the less painful without the words to describe it.

Weeks passed and I neither saw nor heard my son again. What kind of life is this I have lead? Why? What have I done? In my own way, I have asked myself these questions, but can find no answers.

> "Respect existence, or expect resistance!" - Unknown

Four children I have had in this short lifetime. Each one of them has been stolen from me. The regular irritation of plastic tubes against my udder has resulted in sickness and infection on many occasions. My teats are constantly sore, inside I have stomach pains. I feel old although I have only experienced six summers. My milk has run dry and now, after having been driven for several hours in a hot and badly ventilated vehicle, together with many of my sisters, I stand inside a big white building that reeks of anxiety and death. One of my sisters fainted during the journey, and I watched with horror as a human beat her to regain consciousness and forced her to stand up and move. I have also been beaten with a metal rod and have a damaged hind leg. I am barely able to stand erect. I am afraid, I know what is happening here, my intelligence is enough to realise. I can see the stains on the floor and on the aprons of the humans. I can hear distant sisters calling out in such frighteningly horrible manners in neighbouring rooms. I have never heard such intense distressful cries. I stand stupefied and await my fate in dread[42].

It should be noted that although this story may be touching for many, the fate of most cows exploited for milk is in reality far worse. Most of us are completely unaware of what really goes on and how unbearable life for a designated dairy cow truly is. At roughly two years of age they are forcibly impregnated and within twenty four hours of giving birth, their calves are removed, usually slaughtered within the first five days. The mother is left grieving for her lost calf, whilst her milk, which nature intended for her baby, is pumped, pasteurised and sent to supermarket shelves.

Roughly seven weeks later, she will once more be forced pregnant and this cycle will continue until she is no longer able to produce profitable milk quantities. At this point she will herself be murdered, butchered, cooked and gluttonously devoured.

"If the bee disappeared off the surface of the globe, man would have only four years to live".- Albert Einstein.

In Defence of the Bees

Honey is one particular issue that some ethically stanced vegans have disagreements on. The overly sweet nectar syrup has captured the taste buds of many, blinding them of desire to empathise with the plight of bees.

As with pretty much every other ethical issue though, it is normal that mankind attempts to justify his behaviour and it is often reasoned that our relationship with bees is more of a symbiotic one, in that we create for them the comfort and security of their hives, and in exchange the honey is extracted and that the bees will anyway always produce more honey than they themselves actually require.

Without bees this planet would likely be in dire straights, they work hard for their honey and deserve every drop of it. The reality is though, that their hives are systematically seasonally ransacked, often with buckets of cheap sugar water given as a poor substitute[43]. To do this, the bees are often smoked out to make them docile, before their homes are invaded and honey removed.

All we are saying. ♫
Is give bees a chance!

Imagine that you have been working for months, harvesting your own food, then someone comes along and steals it from you. You'd get angry right? You may accuse me of anthropomorphising again, but this is precisely what every other animal will do once their home and livelihood is under threat. They will attempt to defend their home and their well earned food. Any attempt at defence with humans as the aggressor, rarely ends in success. Watch those bees and see if you can find a better emotion than anger to define their moods.

"Let the bee, be"
- Tord Lyseving

Of course, there is no denying that their homes have indeed been crafted specially for them, but everything comes with a price and in this case, the cost is far more than just the stolen honey. The bees are after all unaware of having signed any contract!

The bee populations around the world are currently dying in unprecedented proportions. It is generally suspected that this has to do with the ever increasing use of pesticides (such as the Monsanto flag-ship product Round-Up) and I have no doubt that is partially to blame, but the long term consequences of living in their artificially constructed homes and having their natural food source systematically pillaged from them, often in exchange for something nutritionally inferior, is also playing a major role. Making the species progressively weaker, more intolerant of fluctuations in

Where do bees go
to the bathroom?
At the BP station.

temperature, and more prone and susceptible to disease of many kinds. Back when they were more of an independent insect species, they would build their hive in the hollow of a tree, sure it involved more work for them, but it was the work that nature intended for them and as such, could only be of benefit to them. Such natural hives would have experienced more ranges in temperature, rendering the bee hardier than today's council flatted equivalent.

Being an observant gardener, I too have noticed that there are far less bees than there ever used to be and it is certainly disconcerting to imagine what may happen should the species dwindle yet further. Their role in nature is so crucial to the life of plants that without them the world would be at a loss. Their role needs to be acknowledged and respected and ethically their honey should only really be considered as food should the bees themselves abandon their home in search of further life adventures.

Leave Us Alone!

> "Educating the mind, without educating the heart, is no education at all." - Aristotle

Shod omnivores and fundamentalist veggie-phobes who feel threatened by the vegan movement like to argue for their own rights to eat whatever they choose and to do so without finger pointing or interference. If it were all purely a question of food, they would have every right to protest at any finger pointing, however, they are effectively arguing for *their right to deny the rights of others*. Nobody is physically preventing them from eating the cow, but through their rapacious desires and consumer demands, they are fully denying farmed animals any rights, causing them untold harm and grievance and at the end of their restricted, short, tortured lives, cold blooded murder. And we should stop voicing our disapproval?

Off-the-shelf phrases like "each to their own" prove just how little thought people give to their arguments. The systematic torturing, slaughtering and butchering of animals should not be compared with one's choices in fashion, film, music or religion. The truth of the matter is that one's freedom of choice to eat flesh and other animal products is basically about paying someone else to commit carnage.

Protesters will likely argue that animal killing goes on all around us and that virtually every species participates. Yet, when it comes to human rights, they themselves will likely agree that murder, child molestation, rape, slavery, unwilling prostitution and more

> "People often say that humans have always eaten animals, as if this is a justification for continuing the practice. According to this logic, we should not try to prevent people from murdering other people, since this has been done since the earliest of times" - Isaac Singer

should be policed and prosecuted. And this despite that there are likely examples of much of the above within the behavioural realms of other animal species. Although I agree that we can learn from watching wild animal interaction, I think it rather narrow minded to blatantly assume that their lack of moral conduct justifies our own failing in that regard.

I'd like to point out that marital rape[44] was and in many countries, still is, considered "legal". In fact, it is only within the last fifty years that some countries have begun to criminalise such cases. England not until as late as the 1990s! Many meat eaters would likely object if a rapist were to defend their behaviour as being purely a question of "personal choice" and that others should not impose their moral values on them. To refuse to debate an ethical issue on the grounds that your actions are no one else's business is to fundamentally misunderstand the nature of morality: "These self righteous anti-rapists are so full of themselves, interfering shazbats, should mind their own darned business!". Thus, another demonstration of a popular tactic employed by meat eaters in defence of their supposed freedom of choice; "curses" and "insults". It's always proof that you are winning an argument when you start to get sworn at!

> "There may be times when we are powerless to prevent injustice, but there must never be a time when we fail to protest." - Elie Wiesel

Clearly what is currently legal or illegal is not always an indication of whether or not something is moral or immoral. So just a few years ago, when marital rape was still considered legally acceptable behaviour, those that could see it as unethical were protesting with good cause. Fast forward to today and a vegan, quite similarly, will voice his or her indignation about the unnecessary exploitation and slaughter of sentient beings, even though that too is most clearly fully within legal boundaries!

Everyone is entitled to their own personal tastes, free from interference, but and this shouldn't need saying, **justice** is not a lifestyle choice.

It is also not a question of anyone being "better" than anyone else, another illconceived view that I've heard expressed on more than one occasion. The only person we should be trying to be better than, is ourselves, yesterday.

> Jokes about German sausage are the wurst.

Sense of Humour

I have read and heard, more than once, shod omnivores accusing vegans of having no sense of humour. This is a rather silly accusation based mostly at our unwillingness to laugh, and find funny, sick jokes concerning the suffering of others.

If a serial killer were to joke about his bloodily executed victims, would you seriously find yourself laughing whole heartedly with him? Those poor jokes about the juiciness of a good steak need to be fully grokked. No, I'm not accusing shod omnivores of being serial killers, but I am accusing them of aiding and abetting serial killers in the continuation of their serial killing. Once you've fully grasped the facts, it will be clear just why talking of the deliciousness of bacon is not the least bit comical. Go back further and that bacon was once the flesh on the stomach and back of a living, breathing, sentient, individual being, who, born into misery, likely never knew anything but suffering and torment throughout her entire lifetime, which was macabrely brought short for no other reason than to satisfy the gluttony of shod omnivores. Now laugh!

> Lisa: "I'm going to become a vegetarian"
> Homer: "Does that mean you're not going to eat any pork?"
> Lisa: "Yes"   Homer: "Bacon?"
> Lisa: "Yes Dad"   Homer: "Ham?"
> Lisa: "Dad all those meats come from the same animal"
> Homer: "Right Lisa, some wonderful, magical animal!"

Father Patrick awoke one morning to discover a dead donkey on the front lawn of his house. After examining it and confirming its state, he rang the village police. "Officer, this is Father Patrick here from the local Baptist church. There is a dead donkey on my lawn." The policeman recognising the Irish accent of the priest, decided to joke with him. "Isn't it your job father, to take care of the dead?". The quick witted Irish fellow replied: "Aye, that surely be right officer, but I'm also required to contact the next of kin, see."

Yes, yes. I laughed at The Simpson's[45] quote about the pig (in box to right). but only because it was a shod omnivore joke, not an animal one! It seems many are content with Homer-sapienism as a valid next evolutionary choice. Okay, enough with the

> Animals have voices, open your hearts and hear their cries. If you can't hear them, others will speak for them. If you don't understand them, don't be mad at others for translating. If you ignore their suffering, others have every right to remind you of it. If it were you, bred for the slaughter, would you want people to stop voicing their concern for your suffering, just to give those, who will dine on your carcass a break?

chiropractic mirth; side splitting, rib tickling, ROFLing, and thigh slapping aside, tough issues are raised here, meriting deep reflection and sober consideration.

Dairy Alternatives

So, want to become vegan but can't live without milk? Despair not, supermarkets are full of dairy alternatives, soy and rice milks, soy cheeses, even egg alternatives. Back when I first turned vegan in the 1980s, my wonderful sister and I discovered that flax seeds boiled mildly in water, form into a gooey gluey, egg-like substance, which with further experimentation we found was a perfect substitute as a binder in cake recipes. Of course, I'm not saying any of these foods are ideal (especially not if GMO based!), but at least you'll be able to look a cow and chicken in their eyes and have a clearer conscience. There is NO reason to continue purchasing animal products.

> "Deep within the human constitution lie written laws of nature that should guide man in the conduct of his life."
> - Dr. Herbert M. Shelton

Keep your thoughts positive,
because your thoughts become your words.
Keep your words positive,
because your words become your behaviours.
Keep your behaviours positive,
because your behaviours become your habits.
Keep your habits positive,
because your habits become your values.
Keep your values positive,
because your values become your destiny.
- Gandhi

"If you have men who will exclude any of God's creatures
from the shelter of compassion and pity,
you will have men who will deal likewise
with their fellow men"
- St. Francis of Assisi

"Once you make a decision,
the universe conspires to make it happen."
- Ralph Waldo Emerson

When asked what he thought of Western Civilisation, Gandhi Replied:
"That sounds like a good idea!"

RAW VEGANISM

Go back quarter of a century or less, and the word "vegan" was still virtually unheard of. Finding another vegan in your home town was far from an easy task, and many of us felt quite isolated. In the 1980s I had this small backpack with the slogan "veganism is the way forward" written in bold white letters on it. You'd be surprised how many times people would stop and ask me what it meant. Nowadays things have changed considerably. Nearly everyone in the western world has heard the term, and most people even know, or know of, a vegan or two. The movement has grown substantially, especially since the dawn of the internet, and hooking up with fellow vegans is generally no longer a difficult task.

> "Perhaps the best thing you can do to save the environment, is to eat a plant based diet" - United Nations

Over the past decade or so, the idea of not cooking one's food has also been on the increase, both within the vegan movement, and with the health conscious omnivore populace. For many, the choice to do so is solely one of health and fitness; once one delves deeper into the idea, the health benefits of not cooking become pretty obvious. However, reasons to eat raw, go far beyond matters of physical well-being. I intend to write more on this in following chapters.

It's true, that the cooking process renders many foods edible that otherwise would be rejected raw. Many see this as a blessing, and indeed there may well have been past times of hardship, where pockets of humans would not have survived without these foods. However, those times are over, and it's time we moved on from such sustenance and began to understand the full extent that our diet shapes the world and the ethical role it must inevitably play in preparing for a positive more love filled future.

The ultimate goal of ethics is to refrain from all wrong doing and harm. This is something all true vegans are aware of. It does not mean one cannot or should not break the law, especially not if the law is clearly unjust, but it does mean that we should do our utmost to not cause suffering. With this in mind, it should be clear that we have a duty also to educate ourselves and refrain from practices that harm our own physiological well-beings. We must treat ourselves, our own bodies, as ethically and best we are able. It is our duty to guide and love ourselves, to understand that our bodies are not ours to abuse, but to maintain, nurture and cherish, and use as examples to sway and influence others positively.

For many, the steps from omnivore to vegetarian, and vegetarian to a vegan diet are taken for precisely these reasons. For one's budding desire to improve one's health and consequently life, happiness and longevity.

One's health is clearly a valid reasons for making dietary changes, but unless we can see beyond personal well-being, the

"If your compassion does not include yourself, it is incomplete." - Buddha

likelihood of failure is high. Purely egotistical reasons for change are sadly rarely enough to ensure consistency, and often result in unnecessary and harmful compromises. Eating a fish, for example, because one suddenly feels like it, or sharing the carcass of a turkey because it's thanksgiving and one doesn't wish to upset family. There is no reason for anyone to be upset at another's statement of empathy! Lifelong commitment to dietary change and personal improvement are rarely successful without first broadening one's powers of empathy.

If you do the right thing by all parties concerned (i.e., the fish and the turkeys too), you will also be doing the right thing for yourself! If you wonder about doing the right thing by your host, realise that there is nothing ethically wrong with refusing to eat a meal. If someone gets irrationally upset with this choice, that is purely their issue. Don't let it become yours! If you are consistent with your stance, others will soon accept the decision you have made, even if they don't agree with it.

As mentioned, I intend to get back to ethical issues beyond the duty to one's corporal form, but first I need to explain why and how eating raw is physiologically the right choice.

What did the lettuce say to the celery? - Are you stalking me?

Why Raw?

I'll begin by asking a simple question. What's the furthest you've ever ventured away from human civilization (or "sillyvization", as I prefer calling it, if you'll pardon the bugs-bunnyism)?

I ask this, for if you've ever had opportunity to observe any wild animal, regardless of species, in his natural habitat, you will surely know that all such animals eat their food in its raw, natural state. Human beings, domesticated and feral animals/animals living in close proximity of humans (such as urban foxes), are the only exceptions to this rule. Though, that's not one hundred percent true, as the rule was *species in their natural habitats*, which can hardly said to be the case for little Timmy the cat.

We, on the other hand, are the true omnivores of this planet, eating virtually anything from someone else's fried kidneys, to birds' nests, to piss drenched eggs[46], and chocolate covered grasshoppers[47]. With human ingenuity, there's really little that cannot be rendered palatable[48].

I expressed earlier that we should steer clear of looking up to animals as role models, and generally that's the stance I prefer to take, but in this particular case, I take exception. I really think that human ingenuity has gotten the better of us here. Instead of eating food as nature offers it, we harbour this perverse idea that food should be burnt before consumption, with some people going through life never even tasting anything the way nature intended. Not only has such habit become so ingrained, but also we go about telling everyone how healthy it is too! Believing erroneously that we are doing ourselves an injustice if we don't get at least one cooked meal a day.

> What's on a honeymoon salad? Lettuce alone with no dressing.

At this stage, some readers might be wondering where I am headed with this, and what logic there is behind me stating that such thoughts can be anything resembling erroneous. Bear with me a while, as I intend to get there.

Firstly though, I'd like to point out what I believe to be obvious. Humans are probably the sickest, weakliest, most neurotic species on the globe. Not even the inbred pit bull terriers coming a close second. We have more flavours of dis-ease than one can possibly shake a stick at. Our bodies morph into deformity more and more each day, making us gradually lose our natural born beauty, such that over time we become unrecognisable from how we should look. This may not be clear to those of us who have never given this any thought, because this deformity I talk of is considered relatively "normal" by most; a natural consequence of life and ageing. This is so far from the truth.

In 2010, chronic diseases were the leading causes of death in Australia, with the most common causes including cardiovascular disease, cancer, chronic lower respiratory diseases and diabetes[49]. More than anything else, it is my belief that such ailments are predominantly caused by diet and subjecting one's food to chemical mutating, life shattering heat, prior to consumption. If none of this makes any sense to you, I will now attempt to make it easier to digest.

Organic Food

How many of you go out of your way (or at least feel you perhaps ought to) to obtain organic fruit and vegetables?

Bizarre, perhaps, if one should then return home with them and render them consequently inorganic; Organic also means *pertaining to life*, thus, removing the life force from within a food, easily accomplishable by raising the internal and external temperatures above a certain degree for an extended period of time, will consequently render any food, regardless of how it was grown, inorganic. Hmm, defeating the object somewhat maybe?

> "Food can be a poison or a cure. Why would you choose to ingest toxins when you could be taking the world's best detox medicine. For the purposes of detoxification, let me be clear; always try to eat organic." - Woodson Merrell

The Kitchen as a Chemical Laboratory

Whether we are aware of it or not, the conventional kitchen can be readily compared to a chemical laboratory. Applying heat to a substance is one of the primary methods used in altering its chemical make-up. The chemical structure of all substances changes radically under application of intense heat, a process which inevitably results in destroying all living cells within *any* food subjected to it for long enough. You don't have to stick your hand in a flame, to understand what this means! It will no longer be the natural, energy pulsating, nourishing, life giving substance it once was.

> Every drug that has ever been recalled by the FDA, was first proven to be safe and affective by the FDA.

I have no doubt it is far healthier to eat conventionally grown, chemically sprayed foods, washed and in their raw natural uncooked states, than it is to eat spray free, organic or biodynamically grown foods, cooked.

Picture two carrots, one of them organically grown and cooked, and the other a conventionally grown and thus chemically sprayed one, still raw. What do you think is the difference? Stick them both in the ground and observe. The cooked one will quickly rot, putrefy and grow sludgily mouldy. Whereas there is more than a reasonably good chance that the raw one, despite the chemicals, will live on, sprouting itself a new green leafy carrot top. Similarly, eat the raw one and it will transfer its life giving force to the body, eat the cooked one and it will partially end up as internal gunk. The physiological effects of the chemicals created through the cooking process are *far more proliferous*, thus more harmful, than the conventional ones used while growing the food.

I'm not trying to convince anyone that conventional crops are better than organically grown ones. Far from it, my emphasis here is solely on the folly of rendering organic food inorganic and to make it clearer why cooking is so plainly an unhealthy choice. Of course, if you can source good organic food and leave it organic, i.e., eat it raw, more the better!

> The only person you should try to be better than, is the person you were yesterday.

The Real Cause of Dis-Ease

Unfortunately, our bodies become increasingly addicted to the new chemicals available within these heat modified foods. An addiction that generally lasts from the cradle to the grave. With the grave consequently being reached far quicker than it ought.

Because these foods now contain addictive substances, the body's appetite becomes warped and consequentially, we often eat way in excess of our true needs. Unable to correctly process these biologically reconstructed foodstuffs, to break things down efficiently, the body, over burdened with these inadequately digested residues, consequently becomes latently sick.

These incorrectly absorbed foods, get stored throughout the body as a residue we all know and generally loath with a passion, called..

Mucus

> "They don't think it be like it is but it do"
> - Herman Ree

It matters little how a disease is classified, what Latin name it is cleverly christened, what its symptoms are, where it manifests itself, nor its intensity and severity, there is one culprit whose presence at the scene of the physiological crime is generally predictable, though, perversely enough, widely ignored. It customarily lies sluggishly with few able to recognise the role it has played and rarely gets the finger pointed at it. That miscreant is mucus.

Instead of recognising mucus as the delinquent no-gooder it is, its presence is rarely even acknowledged. The body though, with its own innate wisdom, knows it should not be there and will do its utmost to expel it, from whichever exit point is most readily accessible. As a general rule, this is done through the mouth and nose, but while mucus is sluggishly sludging its way through the blood stream, a simple cut on the knee will suffice for the body to attempt to be rid of it.

Look at that yellow pus oozing its way out of a wound. Compare it with the pus that weeps, honeylike from one's nose during the regular seasonal bout of colds. The difference is minimal and more one of viscosity and consistency than anything else.

Undoubtedly there'll be the occasional forlorn biologist and learned layperson who reading this, will guffaw and protest at my apparent oversimplification, my blatant equalising of mucus and pus, that they know through their microscopes and scientific journals, to be two distinct substances. Put aside the dead leukocytes, glycoproteins, and immunoglobulins though, and one thing that can readily be shown, and that is that on a fully raw diet, the body will not be producing any where near the same quantities of either.

Think of the countless fruitless millions that have been spent to combat common colds and flus. Futile efforts, because the common cold will never be cured, it can only ever be prevented, since the "cold" itself *is* the cure. Prevent the cold and you prevent the onset of virtually every other medical disorder. No more cancers, no more alzheimers (oldtimers). No more hodge-podgkinsons disease.

This may sound far fetched, but the truth is simple and its application and effects, profound.

Germs

Every reaction of the body is a healthy reaction - Your body <u>wants</u> to be in perfect health. Do you?

In retrospect, I am quite baffled as to why I never previously asked myself the very deep question of: "Where does all that mucus come from?". I'll repeat myself, (because it can never be said enough times!). Unable to successfully process third degree burned food, it putrefies and hardens into fat and is dispersed throughout one's body. At times it is released as a mucus slime, becoming the ideal home and terrain for germs and bacteria to thrive within.

Contrarily, allopathic medicine would have us believe that colds are caused by invisible little airborne sprites. Microscopic beings that invade our bodies causing us untold discomfort. Not altogether antithetic to primitive thinking that the devil takes possession of you. The medical establishment would have us believe lots of things.

How fully we have accepted the explanation of imperceptible burrowing beings. But prepare yourself for something alternative, something profound. Are you ready for it? Grasp the sides of your chair. *Germs can only survive if the terrain for them to thrive in is already present.*

> "What the sick need are teachers not treaters, health schools not hospitals, instruction not treatment, education in right living not training the sick habit. Both they and their advisors must get rid of the curing idea and the practices built up thereon." - Herbert M. Shelton

It is rather like having a dirt encrusted dustbin, infested with flies. From the medical industries perspective, the flies are the nuisance and must be combated and destroyed. They prescribe fly killer, which once sprayed inside the dustbin will kill the flies, leaving the dustbin to rot in its own filth. After a while, other flies will arrive, or cockroaches, or more. If the bin is never cleaned, no amount of pesticides will ever see it truly clean. The superfly will forever mutate and finds its way back home!

Similarly, while mucus is ever present, things will find their home within it. Cosy warm and sludgy. Yippee!

In fact, the germs, like the flies, are really doing us a favour. Although irritating, they do serve to slowly but surely clean away the decay and with each batch of germs, the body with renewed vigour, will try its darnedest to eradicate the mucus within which they breed. The idea of simply repressing this eradication is frankly, unreservedly ludicrous.

> My doctor told me to avoid any unnecessary stress, so I didn't open his bill.

You would be grossly mistaken if you were to believe that this is a new idea, one that I've just concocted. It has been recognised since the days of Louis Pasteur, the guy who came up with the rather sick idea of pasteurising stuff. Although his proposition has widely sunken into obscurity, some time after the middle of the 19th century, Antoine Béchamp, a contemporary biologist of Pasteur, came up with the theory that it was the terrain which was the real issue needing to be addressed. In his own words: 'Le microbe, *c'est rien*, le *milieu*, c'est tout' - 'The germ *is nothing*, the environment (it thrives in) *is everything*'. Pasteur and Béchamp were largely in disagreement and competition with one another over this. However, on his deathbed, Pasteur finally recanted, saying that Béchamp had been right all along, and that *the terrain was indeed everything.*

However, I'm guessing that since germ theory was seen as being financially far more lucrative a venture, far more profitable, the pharmaceutical industry has chosen to fully dismiss his final testimony as the insanity of a dying man. Would that we all should suffer such insanity!

Hereditary Issues

One might contend that certain issues are hereditary and thus ineludible. One has to understand though, that the body is like a finely tuned piece of machinery. It needs high quality oil to keep it running at optimum efficiency. Start feeding it low grade oil, and any dirt flecks and impurities within that oil will get caught up and accumulate at the weakest spots within the machine. This is why people apparently suffer from different indispositions. On the surface it may look like the guy with the dodgy knee, and the guy with the heart problem are experiencing completely separate issues, but the reality is that the sufferings of both are profoundly connected. Hereditary issues are nothing more than inherent "weak points" passed on from generation to generation. By re-adopting healthy living habits, they can quite easily be avoided.

Digestion and Assimilation

"I began to wonder why we cuddle some animals and put a fork in others." - Henry Spira

Physiologically, the anatomical body is generally occupied with one of these four activities: Digestion, Assimilation, Elimination and Healing, and generally speaking, although all four are regularly in process somewhat simultaneously, Digestion and Assimilation take precedence.

I think we all understand the role of each of these two: Digestion being the process by which food consumed/ingested is broken down into absorbable microscopical elements, and Assimilation being the process by which those elements are then reassembled and incorporated within the body.

Because we eat the wrong things, and often way in excess, these two processes generally take up more time than they should, thus impeding the other anatomical functions where they are put on the back burner and momentarily neglected.

Elimination

Without the required constant flow of elimination, the body will become, for want of a better term, burdened, or increasingly more toxic. This is more than just intestinal constipation, as the internal waste needing evacuation is stored all throughout the body, and it is this gradual increase in toxicity which causes the undermining of our healths, for our bodies to become deformed, misshapen, puffed up and for one's natural beauty to inevitably wane. It's sort of the opposite to the H.C. Anderson story, where we all start out as beautiful swans, but after being slapped, prodded, poked, kneaded, stuffed, puffed, bulged and corrupted, we end up as uncomely ducklings.. (perhaps *dumplings* would be more appropriate than *ducklings*. Ugly duckling is an oxymoron, two words that basically contradict each other, rather similar to "military intelligence").

> "Instead of worrying about what could go wrong, change your thoughts to what could go right. When you change the negative thought into a positive one, it eliminates the negative one." - Roy T. Bennett

Predominantly, normal elimination involves basic usage of the intestinal and urinal tracts with the kidneys acting as filters. This process on a healthy diet is generally smooth and trouble free and should be altogether void of any discomfort. Because of our warped sense of what constitutes food though, and because elimination is frequently postponed indefinitely, other major elimination organs are called into play.

Detox

You don't have to be a brain surgeon to understand it, just a rocket scientist (only kidding)!

> Detox is your friend. NOT your enemy.

Eradication of internal filth, detoxification or simply *detox* by which it is commonly referred, is a sort of emergency elimination. It occurs when the body, with its own innate wisdom, decides to slow down other tasks, and instead concentrate the bulk of its efforts on elimination. It is generally accompanied by a consequential loss of appetite, such that the body can stop digestion and assimilation, and focus purely on the much required elimination and ultimately healing (more on this soon).

Some of the more common symptoms of detox, are nausea, headaches, stomach cramps, dizziness, blocked sinuses and much more. The common cold is probably the most common form of major detox the body regularly initiates, without it, internal affairs would become increasingly more serious, it may even become so saturated with toxins, that a sudden keel over and die scenario would not eventually be out of the question. It is generally unwise to attempt to suppress detox through supposed medicine or pills or any other method and important to understand that it is a normal healthy bodily reaction. Your body knows well what it is doing, trust it, don't try and fight it. Contrarily, one should rejoice that the body functions so well, and that its internal wisdom demands time out to cleanse itself.

So, although we inevitably feel horrible, miserable and negative throughout the detox experience, in reality we are getting better.

Don't despair, be aware!

"The shorter the chain between raw food and fork, the fresher it is and the more transparent the system is." - Joel Salatin

Although germs may be present during detox and seemingly compounding the issue, they are not the enemy, in fact they often serve to provoke one's physiology to go into a (beneficial) detox mode. Again, making a comparison to something external from biology, it is like a house full of mess and dustballs desperately in need of a good spring clean. It may be the case that the occupant is just too lazy to undertake the clean, but introduce a plague of cockroach or mice and suddenly there is increased motivation to tidy. Similarly, the germs need not even be present. The body may just decide there is too much internal filth and begin detox, regardless of the presence of pestilence. This is why you can move into a cabin out in the wilderness, far away from the city and any of its bugs and even though there are no microbes present, one can still catch a cold!

I hope my little analogies can be forgiven, because here's another one: Let us imagine for a second, that there is a little worker whose job it is to break up 25 cardboard boxes an hour. The boxes are crisp and clean and it's not a tiresome task. It's an easy job and the little man is happy doing it and can do so indefinitely, day in and day out.

"If you are going through hell, keep going." - Winston Churchill

Let us suppose now, that the little man starts being given 30 boxes an hour. Suddenly he can't keep up any more. And what's worse, these 30 boxes are no longer crisp and clean, they are dirty, soiled, hot and sticky. The little man gets overwhelmed by it all. He tries his best to keep up, but ends up having to store decaying half broken down cardboard boxes all around him. In the end, he has so many encircling him, that he has to shout *stop*! He needs a rest.

This is called a healing crisis. The little man is our body and the cardboard boxes are what we eat. The crisp fresh ones, are the food that nature intended for us, unadulterated by heat, the dirty soiled ones, are cooked foodstuffs and the putrefying discarded half broken down ones, are the mucus. Once there are too many half broken boxes within us, we have to stop. We have to become sick (= we have to clean ourselves!) Then the mucus starts coming out from everywhere. We have cardboard boxes flowing out of our ears and from every available orifice. (NOTE: This is an analogy, don't confuse cardboard boxes with cardboard hydrates, - actually you'd think it should be cardboard dehydrates?).

> "A man can live and be healthy without killing animals for food; therefore, if he eats meat, he participates in taking animal life merely for the sake of his appetite." - Leo Tolstoy

If you can genuinely understand why it is, that the body requests detox, then you are, in theory at least, really more than halfway toward freeing yourself from regular bouts of detox. All you then need to do is act upon that knowledge!

Major Detox Points

Here are the major points to consider concerning detox:

1. Detox is a good thing, never your enemy.
2. Detox is never pleasant.
3. Detox can take on many different and varied forms and guises.
4. Detox can be sped up (and intensified!) by not eating! (see Fasting, below)
5. Future detox can be vastly prevented (by changing one's habits), but it is generally wise to not hinder present detox.
6. All consumed cooked foods, will (eventually/sooner or later) be the cause of some detox.
7. Detox can sometimes appear to be ongoing. Especially if you eat a high percentage of raw vegan foods and small amounts of cooked foods.
8. Most forms of dis-ease from which we suffer are predominantly some form of detox or other, or a result of the

lack of such.

9. Detox is the body's way of cleansing itself as it strives toward optimum health.

10. Detox is initiated for two main reasons. Either because the body decides that it is in desperate need of a "spring clean", or because the body is invaded by an external menace (that incidentally, can only survive and thrive where filth is already present).

11. Remember. Your headache is not caused by lack of aspirin in your diet!

Cancer

"Truth, like gold, is to be obtained not by its growth, but by washing away from it all that is not gold." - Leo Tolstoy

As we age and continue making the same dietary mistakes, elimination is often postponed indefinitely. Decades of eating the wrong foods and the consequent enormous backlog requiring elimination, ultimately leads to more serious complications. Cancer being one of the most popular and feared afflictions.

Perversely enough, billions of dollars continue to be spent on cancer research. Sausage sizzles and cake-stands are set up to raise money for the cause, with apparently zero recognition that it is precisely the sizzling sausages and the refined sugar and wheat cakes, that are part and parcel of the problem erroneously trying to be cured. Yes, cancer is no more something that can ever truly be cured than is the common cold. It can only be prevented and if the right habits are adopted, the body will rid itself of the cancer, which is precisely why fasting and healthy changes to one's lifestyle, have been known to heal patients suffering from all manner of ailments. No! All we have to do is stop feeding the cancer and it will naturally disappear of its own accord! What's that? You don't believe there is a connection between diet and cancer? Although science has yet to realise the full extent that diet and cancer are related, it is slowly beginning to see the truth[50].

I believe that while the cause of cancer lies mostly unaddressed, no investigation and research into T-cells will ever amount to anything of lasting purpose. Researchers may be increasing human understanding of physiology, but in terms of combating cancer, they are effectively barking up the wrong tree. In fact, the three conventional treatments for cancer, chemotherapy, radiation treatment and surgery have all been shown to instigate cancer when performed on an otherwise seemingly healthy body! Having trouble believing this, please see this informative video[51] with Dr. Glidden who explains quite clearly that chemotherapy doesn't work in 97% of cases! With this in mind, it seems to me that such treatments are more about squeezing more money out of the system than actually healing anyone[52]. In my opinion, I think diagnosis often compounds the problem, and many people would live longer not knowing they had cancer and could heed the uncommon sense I share here, rather than being diagnosed and seeking conventional treatment for it.

Here is one man's testimony to curing his own cancer[53].

Fasting

> Fasting doesn't mean eating fast food!

When we transit from the standard cooked food diet of zombie flesh and stodgy lasagne dumpling pies, or whatever it is one eats, onto a lighter diet, (whether it be vegetarian, vegan, raw food, or especially a fully fledged fruitarian one), detox is pretty much inevitable. Any such transition should give the body a reprise. An ease back on digestion and assimilation, such that the body can turn its concentration toward elimination. If we desire however to really speed things up, fasting is a sure fire way of rapidly bringing on detox.

If undertaken correctly, it is about the closest one can get to a true "cure all", except if you can truly fathom what's happening, you'll know what a misnomer that is. Once one understands that the body is constantly struggling toward perfect health, and that the only thing preventing it from attaining such an ideal state, is our minds and the bad habits that we have embraced and adopted, health will return of its own accord. Wagging its tail behind it.

Often simply skipping a meal or two will suffice for its repercussions to begin. Digestion and assimilation will trickle slowly to a halt, leaving elimination to finally take the helm and kick in at full throttle. In fact, this is sure proof that one's body is in a toxic state. A truly normal healthy body should easily be able to skip a meal or two without any discomfort.

> What does a clock do when it's hungry? It goes back four seconds.

Fasting opens up the proverbial can of worms that the body so desperately needs to rid itself of. Once elimination is under way, discomfort **will**, sooner or later, be experienced, this has nothing to do with the body starving as is often

70

supposed. It is simply a sign of the body being toxic and of those toxins being released into the blood stream for elimination!

Fasting does however have its drawbacks and unless you are totally sure you are up confident and up for the experience, I wouldn't recommend it to anyone without supervision.

The problems with fasting are the internal demons. And I'm not referring to the germs this time! For most it will, initially at least, be a constant struggle. Cravings will rear their ugly heads and resisting them will be a genuine challenge. Once you decide to break the fast, although there is a right way to do so, easing one's way slowly back into foods, through juices first etc., many will find the urge to binge irresistible, often undoing whatever good work has otherwise been accomplished.

For this reason, it may be easier, with milder detox symptoms, to go on a fresh fruit juice cleansing cure instead.

Juice Feasting[b]

"Don't let yesterday, take up too much of today." - Will Rogers

Whenever someone talks of doing a juice fast, or fasting on watermelon, or fasting on grapes they are, semantically speaking, fooling themselves. The term *juice fasting* is another classic example of an oxymoron. Think about it, many of us may actually break-fast (the first meal of the day after a night of not eating) on a glass of grapefruit juice, or a bunch of grapes. So with that in mind, it hardly should be considered that a week on orange juice is actually fasting. You would be breaking (the) fast with each glass you took!

"The highest form of ignorance is when you reject something you don't know anything about." - Wayne Dyer

There is a vast distinction between fasting and going on a juice cure, or juice feast.

Fasting requires that one takes no foods, solid or liquid. Only water is permitted (unless one dry fasts, which is even more fierce!), on the other hand, on a juice feast one is never fasting, but can drink as much juice as one feels comfortable with.

By making this distinction, I am not trying to undermine the benefits that can be gained from juice feasting. they are somewhat similar to

---

b   Some years back, I coined the term "juice feasting" - I liked it because it was just that little "e" (f(e)asting) that made the difference and since then, I'm happy to notice how the term has definitely been gaining in popularity.

fasting, only radically less intense. In theory there is no reason why one cannot go on a juice feast indefinitely, especially if a wide range of fresh juices are consumed and enough of them to cover one's needs.

I realise there is a great deal more that could be said on the subject of both fasting and juicing and recommend those interested to read up more elsewhere. I think you might find Herbert Shelton's work on Fasting and Sunbathing quite inspiring. It can be read online for free here[54].

How long does detox take?

During my years as a fruitarian, I have been asked on numerous occasions how long one can expect detox to go on for. This is rather like the proverbial question "how long is a piece of string" and there really is no straight forward answer.

How long it will take to get totally clean will be different for each individual, taking from just weeks for some, and many months or possibly even years, for others. It will all depend on age and state of health and living environment, the quality of the food eaten and surely other factors that are too numerous to mention. As a rule of thumb, the younger and healthier one is, the easier and smoother things should flow and the quicker the benefits should be visible.

> Two Christians were lost in the desert. One named Nigel, the other Pete. They were dying of hunger and thirst when they suddenly came upon an oasis, with what looked like a mosque in the middle.
> Nigel said to Pete : "Look, let's pretend we are Muslims, otherwise we'll not get any food or drink. I am going to call myself Mohammed."
> Pete refused to change his name, he said: "My name's Pete and I will not pretend to be someone else".
> The Imam of the mosque received both well and asked about their names.
> Nigel said: "My name is Mohammed."
> Pete said : "My name is Pete. "
> The Imam turned to the helpers of the mosque and said:
> " Please bring some food and water for Pete"
> Then he turned to the other and said : "Well Mohammed I hope you are aware that we are still in the holy month of Ramadan."

To make it more clear what you actually have to contend with, I would like to refer to a story Morris Krok mentioned in one of his books. I have several of his books in storage on the other side of the globe, so am unable to confirm in which of them the story was told, but believe it was likely in "Fruit the Food"[55]. If anyone can verify please do tell me. Anyhow, I'll probably get chastised for citing a story from memory that I'm unable even to recall which book it was from, but here goes nothing.

Morris had been on a predominantly fruitarian diet for some years. I recall he wrote that he was in good physical health and was running marathons on a pretty regular basis, often travelling around his country (South Africa) to attend different organised marathons.

On one particular occasion, he travelled to a town and checked in to a room at a motel or hotel in preparation for a marathon due to begin the following morning. That evening, while relaxing in his room, someone knocked at his door.

Morris got up to see who was there and to his surprise, a woman he had not seen for many years stood in front of him. If memory serves correct, I believe she was an old flame. She'd heard that Morris was in town, and had decided to pay him an impromptu visit. Morris invited her in.

Not wanting to arrive empty handed however, she had taken a bar of chocolate along with her and not just any old bar, mind, but a particular brand that she knew was (or had once been) a favourite of Morris's.

Now Morris was taken aback and pleasantly surprised to see a familiar face in an unfamiliar setting and for whatever reason or excuse he may have given himself, he decided to share the chocolate with his friend. Together they slowly polished off the chocolate bar while reminiscing on bygone days.

Now, on to the result. And this is pretty profound, so I really hope you are all sitting alert and comfortably and are able to all learn something from it. Brace yourself!

The following morning, Morris awoke with terrible cramps. I think in his legs, but they may have also been in his stomach. So

> "It is okay to doubt what you have been taught to believe." - Unknown

severely it affected him, that he was not only unable to run the marathon he had intended, but also he recalls that it took him one whole week before he had fully recovered and was feeling his normal fit self again!

So think about that. If it can take a healthy body one whole week to

73

recover from just half a bar of chocolate, imagine how long it will take for a body to recover from twenty, thirty, forty or fifty years of constant dietary disaster onslaught?.

In the Edmond Szekely book on fasting[56], the story is told of Jesus (supposedly an Essene, thus by some definitions, borderline Fruitarian with his dietary wisdom), who took people into the wilderness to fast. There he told them, that for each year they had sinned and indulged in eating impure foods, they would have to fast for one day to recover. Thus a forty year old, to regain the given birth right of health, would need to fast for forty days.

> Blaming someone else for the cold you *catch* is ignorant denial. You're avoiding responsibility for your own bad habits.

Of course, this was just a rule of thumb and in today's more hi-tech society, with its car exhaust fumes, chemicals in and on everything, and its excessively degenerative, denatured, greasy, fast food, burger pizza fried lard, pasta salted sugar concoctions, I have no doubt that this basic rule of 'one day for each year' would no longer be remotely workable in the harsh stodgy reality of 21st century gastronomy.

And of course, too, this was a rule of thumb while fasting, which as I've stated is probably the most intense form of cleansing the body can undergo, leaving the body with little choice other than to fully focus on detox, elimination and the inevitable healing that comes with such.

So back on a juices, raw vegan diet, or fruitarian diet, how long do you expect it'll take to fully liberate oneself from previous flaws in one's diet? How long do you think it might take before those erred foods finally finish their influence upon us?

Of course, there is no single answer to this question. It would all depend on one's age, state of health, environment and more. The answer may vary greatly from individual to individual, but I'm afraid one thing is for sure, most people tend to quit far in advance of the light at the end of the tunnel.

> On the back of a cigarette packet I stumbled upon, it said that for annual causes of death in Australia, 203 are due to murders, 863 due to illegal drugs, 1,731 to motor vehicle accidents and 19,019 due to tobacco related issues. I would love to see how many more deaths there are that are food related, I am sure the number would far outweigh the mere 19,000 cigarette deaths!

They walk away, disheartened and disillusioned, believing their newly chosen diet is to blame for their apparently waning health; unaware that in order to get better, the road is tough and all manner of physical ailments may befall us.

We all need to understand the true impact that the conventional diet will have on our frail physiologies. Actually, I take that back, I think our physiologies are far from frail, given the abuse they are somehow miraculously able to withstand over the average course of a lifetime.

Recounting from my own life experience, I recall that after vagabonding my way south, from Norway to the French Pyrénées (an event that took me approximately one year and five thousand kilometres on my push-bike), I settled for a while in a French Community called "Douceur et Harmonie[57]". On arriving, I fully believed in, and tried my utmost to practice, the fruitarian philosophy, but was met with a good deal of opposition there.

I admit, I have no real problem understand their scepticism, as very clearly at the time, I was still regularly battling cooked food addiction, while otherwise struggling to live on a raw vegan, predominantly fruit diet. The consequences? Well, I was pretty much constantly detoxing and thus was undoubtedly far from being the great vision of health I so desperately desired to be. I also had a couple of other major health issues that the universe threw at me and although both were completely unrelated to the fruit diet, the severity of them sent the community into panic mode, believing my lack of culinary wisdom would be the death of me.

> If you give up, it means you never *really* wanted it.

I reckon this was the only time in my life, that I've ever experienced anything that was bordering on depression. Probably due to the ever present detox, my emotions were pretty turbulent at the time, and I was often experiencing anger too.

Thankfully, I eventually had the determination enough to move on with my life and pursue my destiny. I see everything that has happened to me to be significant in some way, and praise be to the great white spirit, that despite any hardships that I've endured, I've managed through it all to stay focused on what I believe is right, and despite that my own journey to fruit took so many years, it is truly joyous to be here and to know that the path is forever unfolding.

So please, please don't expect to see immediate bright and shining health. A sound understanding and a great deal of self patience will likely first be required!

Enemas and Laxatives

Patience is one of those frequently lacking virtues that will cause some to seek out ways to speed up the detox process. Colon cleanses through the likes of enemas and laxatives are two such methods frequently turned to. On the surface such procedures may seem harmless enough, with the effects soon made obvious, however they should be avoided at all cost. Once you have stopped polluting your body with the lower foods, especially the animal cadavers and cooked breads etc., detox will occur naturally at its own rightful pace. Speeding things up by such methods will likely result in weakening the natural workings of the body, making them lazy and dependent on them. Raw foods and plenty of juices may be slower, but even the most stubbornly encrusted mucoid plaques will slowly dissolve and eventually dislodge themselves from the walls of the intestines. Let nature take its own course!

Healing

Rather like elimination, healing, the fourth of the body's internal tasks, often gets postponed due to the ever present digestion and assimilation

"Look deep into nature, and then you will understand everything better." - Albert Einstein

demanded by a body given inferior food choices. In many ways, elimination and healing are deeply entwined with one another and once elimination is under way, so too is healing. However, besides healing from the ravages of toxins and excess mucus, there is another kind of healing that regularly also gets delayed. I am referring, of course, to cuts, sprains, strains, twists, pulled muscles, bruises and more.

If one is eating well and living well, healing from such wounds should be relatively quick and none too objectionable. True one may not be able to entirely prevent pain, but it can certainly be minimised. If, on the other hand, one eats a more conventional diet, the reverse is true. Healing is abated and the level of pain experienced often increases dramatically.

There are cases of scars that having been there for decades, suddenly heal after one has made positive improvements to one's food intake. I recall Arnold Ehret, who wrote in one of his books[58], about a friend of his that after walking for an extended period in the mountains, breathing clean fresh air and living on predominantly grapes, experienced an almost miraculous healing of a lifelong affliction of stuttering.

I also once had a badly injured ankle, which, months later, after finally healing for the most, left me with a slight limp. Part of me resigned myself to what seemed like the fact, that I would likely never have full usage of it again. However, after some days of water fasting and the accompanying detox which had quickly reared its ugly head, jamming its gnarled clubbed foot in the door, my ankle suddenly became bathed in warmth. Half an hour later, to me surprise and pleasure, all movement had returned, and my ankle had completely healed.

> "The pharmaceutical industry does not create cures, it creates customers." - Unknown

What we eat not only effects us physically, but also mentally and behaviourally. This has been demonstrated quite effectively by prisons that have adopted vegan diets for inmates, resulting in, profound changes of social demeanour[59]. Similarly, psychiatric hospital patients have also been shown to benefit from being fed vegetarian diets. I would love to see what could be accomplished if such institutions adopted raw vegan or, better yet, fruitarian diets!

The Medical Industry

Although I wouldn't do away with it entirely, because I do believe they do an otherwise good job in the emergency ward. Putting people back together after serious injuries, stitches, realignments and helping set fractured or broken bones and all that sort of stuff, that's about as far as my allegiance to them goes. Outside of the ER, I see the industry as a whole as little more than a glorified institution of legalised drug pushers, employed by the state to do just that; push drugs, peddling their wares on a public that worships them in an often godlike fashion. If a doctor says something's true, it unquestionably must be!

> "We now live in a nation where doctors destroy health, lawyers destroy justice, universities destroy knowledge, governments destroy freedom, the press destroys information, religion destroys morals and our banks destroy the economy." - Chris Hedges

In training to be a doctor, it is often the case that very little emphasis is placed on the study of nutrition[60]. In fact, only thirty percent of

77

medical schools in the U.S. require a separate nutrition course, and on average, students received 23.9 contact hours of nutrition instruction during medical school[61]. It is clear from these figures that the industry as a whole directs little attention toward diet and the role it plays in health.

It seems pretty obvious to me that most issues people want resolving, when they go to visit their local GPs, have their roots in bad diet. As such, a wise course of action would surely be for a doctor to examine the diet and lifestyle of a patient and prescribe changes to it. This should be clear to all concerned, just by looking at the warped body shape of the patient. Instead of being slim and agile, they are malformed and stiffly jointed, with waists, hips and more bulging at the seams! My own experience with doctors has shown me that many of them suffer the same afflictions. I question how we can place our trust in anyone to heal us, who does not understand enough about health to maintain their own.

> "Let go of thoughts that do not make you stronger." - Unknown

Instead of making patients aware of their questionable dietary practices, GPs will generally shepherd you into their little offices, look at the symptoms of whatever it is that is making you feel uncomfortable, allocate some complex Latin name to it and prescribe some kind of toxic substance to suppress those symptoms. Effectively bashing them on the head. Outside of possibly other drugs, alcohol or cigarettes and advice to cut down on the fried and fatty foods, rarely is it the case that they will tell you to change your habits. Habits that many doctors are themselves hooked on. The medication they prescribe will seriously not do anything to improve your condition long term. More likely it will end up hastening your journey toward an early funeral[62].

This is the reason why it is ultimately of great benefit to patients when doctors go on strike. Statistics show that whenever doctors and the medical industry have done so, the mortality rate in the affected area has fallen dramatically.

During doctors strikes:

In Bogata, Colombia, in 1976, the death rate fell by thirty five percent. In LA, California, in

> If it were *you*, faced with the injustice; the unfair incarceration, the fattening and abattoir destiny. What argument would you consider reasonable to make such a life acceptable to you?

1976 the death rate dropped eighteen percent. In Israel, 1973, the death rate dropped fifty percent. Only once before was there a similar drop in Israel and that was during a previous doctors strike in the beginning of the 1950s. After each strike, the death rate jumped again to its normal level[63].

They apparently have little, to no real clue to the real causes of human physiological discomfort, or dis-ease and seem to be working under the warped logic that a headache is solely due to lack of aspirin intake. In reality, although admittedly not immediately obvious, it is as if someone keeps banging their head against a wall, and then goes to the doctor to get headache pills. Bizarre. To say the least.

A few years back, we had this next door neighbour who was morbidly obese. With the aid of crutches she could barely walk ten meters without sweating profusely, puffing and wheezing and feeling overwhelmed with exhaustion. I paid her a visit one day and proposed that I might begin making her a fresh juice daily. (this woman appears in our documentary *Pure fruit*[1].)

Surprisingly she agreed to the proposal and from that day forth, I began administering her with the said juice, mostly fruit based, but sometimes she had carrot, celery and other vegetables too. And pretty large quantities of it! A couple of litres of fresh juice daily! In fact, I'd estimate, that she was drinking more fresh juice than either Květa and I do, on the days when we just take juice and nothing else.

Nature is cheaper than therapy!

Of course, she was still eating all the other stuff she does, the breads and meats and beefy, greasy, fry up, roasted, lamb buttocky things, which despite her immobility she somehow managed to extraordinarily prepare for herself in her small council flat apartment.

The juices were most definitely beneficial. Despite the fact that she still overate other stuff that clearly wasn't lessening her burden, she one day happily reported that she had begun more regular bowel movements and claimed to be eating less as the juice had replaced her in-between meals, or at least some of them. To an extent.

On two consecutive hospital visits, over a four month period, she discovered on both occasions that she had lost two kilograms in weight. Okay. Not a great deal as a percentage of her overall weight, but as she had never before been seen to lose any weight at her regular six to eight week weigh ins, those four kilos were enough for her to understand that the juices were definitely a good thing in her life.

I recall carrying her juice through to her one morning, and finding her sick with the flu and pounding headaches. (Her first major detox in ages and most definitely a positive sign that her body was improving). She'd just gotten back from a trip to her doctor, who had, ever-so-wiselyʕᶜ, prescribed her a course of antibiotics. It's likely there are some readers that will miss out on the profundity of that!

This, together with whatever other medications she was on, and the occasional trips in an ambulance for heart or other obesity related dilemmas she had over the course of many years inflicted upon herself, must have been costing her, or someone, a small fortune.

> "The doctor of the future will give no medicine but will interest his patients in the care of the human frame, in diet and in the cause and prevention of disease." - Thomas Edison

Clearly the establishment had no desire for her to get better, as she was undoubtedly one of their best customers. Had the goal been to genuinely help the poor lady, rehab would have been suggested or even enforced, where she would have been treated like others with obvious addiction problems. (Since we moved out from that particular living accommodation, and moved up to our beloved tropical home, we have no idea what became of her).

Looking back at that time, I realise how almost comical it is, that of all the "treatment" she received, the only thing that was genuinely giving her any real benefit, was her daily juices and perversely enough, other than the cost of the raw ingredients, the only thing she was getting for free.

> "The most useful asset of a person is not a head full of knowledge, but a heart full of love, with ears open to listen, eyes open to see and hands willing to help." - Unknown

Recently the news featured another case of lunacy that caught my eye. An obese American woman had consulted her doctor, about an on going case of particularly troublesome body odour. Apparently she smelt so badly that she had lost all her friends and no one would even sit next to her on public transport or the bingo hall. How did the doctor solve this clearly embarrassing dilemma? He arranged surgery to have her sweat glands removed! The same kind of idiocy is routinely recommended for those suffering inflamed tonsils. And these people have PhDs! If I

---

c   For those of you unfamiliar with this punctuation mark: ʕ it is a "percontation point", used to indicate there is another layer of meaning to a sentence.

were unaware of the financial incentive behind such procedures, I'd be inclined to believe that they were educated far beyond their intelligence.

Okay, okay, I may be excessively over-generalising somewhat, it should be clear that there are many well meaning, knowledgeable, open minded individuals that have made it their life choice to work within the health care industry. I admittedly sometimes get carried away with the negative side of the drug trade. To the undoubtedly many, good positive people that genuinely care for those that need it, I acknowledge your presence, and mean you no disrespect.

In essence though I stand by the crux of what I am saying and believe that once one has learned to eat properly, doctors and their diagnosis of ailments combined with the chemical addressing of symptoms, will eventually be a thing of the past.

> "Great spirits have always encountered violent opposition from mediocre minds." - Albert Einstein

Additional Benefits

In addition to the health improvements one can confidently expect to experience if switching to a raw vegan diet, there are other perks to a raw regime. I intend going into these in more detail in following chapters, but think of that extra kitchen space you'll gain when you no longer need that bulky oven, the electricity you'll save when you no longer have to cook, and the money you'll save when you no longer need all those pots and pans and detergents to rid them of those ingrained grease, slime, burn stains.

> "Cutting out bad habits is far more effective than cutting out organs." - Dr. Herbert M. Shelton

Grain

I look at bread as being an iconic symbol of much that is wrong with cooked foodstuffs throughout most regions of this planet. Of course, the mutilated animal corpses, fish cadavers, dairy sludge and imprisoned birds exploited for their eggs, are far worse in terms of what they are doing to ours and others' bodies, but this fact does little to lessen the crime of bread and rice and other grains.

Grain is the summit. the ever-present daily staple of shod vegetarian/vegan and zombie flesh eating omnivores alike. It is the most unnatural of all vegan/vegetarian foods, highly environmentally destructive and generally inedible without tedious prior preparations.

81

Its production is extremely labour intensive and its monocrop necessity, causes widespread environmental destruction. Were you to be presented with a handful of grain plus a few peanuts and given the task of preparing your very own peanut butter sandwiches from scratch, (i.e., growing your own wheat and peanuts, caring for them, weeding them, harvesting them etc.) you would undoubtedly think twice before agreeing to the challenge.

The whole idea of monocrops goes against the grain of nature. Look at a field of grass, you might think it's just grass, but this would be a most inaccurately casual observation. In reality the field will likely contain, at bare minimum, many tens of different types of plant species, sometimes the variety will be within the hundreds. That's what nature is all about, diversity. Any attempt to forcibly eradicate that diversity, as is the necessity when growing wheat or any other kind of grain, battles against nature, requiring either intense manual labour, or a potent smorgasbord of chemicals; herbicides, pesticide and their ilk.

Not only is the production of grain slowly destroying our beautiful home planet, its baked consumption is one of the most common addictive foodstuffs out there and possibly the most major mucus forming food eaten daily. Once your body is clean enough, all it takes is one or two mouthfuls of bread to recognise its quick and silent bodily phlegmification.

If you are going to eat grain, which as an Eden Fruitarian I don't endorse at all, but nevertheless recognise that at times they may be the better of choices, then consider instead of baking them first, to sprout them in soil and harvest the green shoots for juicing instead.

Teaching our children not to step on bugs, is as valuable to the children as it is to the bugs.

Salt

I do not believe the body has anything to gain from its consumption. On the contrary, I see salt intake as detrimental to longevity. As stated earlier, physiologically, the human body is well adapted for processing organic, "living" food and transforming it into the fuel the body needs in order to survive and maintain health. As it is inorganic, salt is no more a food than is dirt or rock dust. It is solely an appetite stimulator and serves no real purpose other than to promote gluttony and excessive drinking. Plants are rich in minerals that they are able to absorb from the earth and sunlight. Minerals in plants are not identical to minerals in the earth, sand, rock or sea water, as they have been converted by the plant to an organic state by the miraculous powers of nature, and thus they are contrarily well suited to our bodies.

I remember as a kid always being told that we had to eat salt, that it was a necessity, when we run around working or playing, we sweat, and the sweat contains salt, and that consequently such salt must be replaced. Back in the day, before discovering the benefits of eating raw, I bought into this theory, and the truth is that when I began consuming less salt, I suffered on occasion from leg cramps, labouring under the belief that these cramps were due to insufficient salt intake, I would often eat salted potato crisps in an effort to eliminate them. Indeed, it did appear as if by doing so, the agony of cramp I suffered would lessen. However I now see more clearly, that it was likely the salt that was causing the cramps in the first place, being more of a "cold turkey" after affect than a genuine body cry for a life giving necessity. In any case, anything the body expels through the skin or anywhere else, it does so because the stuff should not be in there!

> "It is always a much easier task to educate uneducated people than to re-educate the mis-educated."
> - Dr. Herbert M Shelton

Superfoods

I mentioned earlier about the raw food's movement being hijacked by charlatans out to make a fast buck. "Superfoods" are one of their best money spinners. They sell blue green algae (basically pond scum), dried wheat grass, maca powder, raw cacao, marine phytoplankton (basically whale fodder) and shrivelled goji berries to name but a small handful of their wares. In my opinion this is nothing more than a money making scam and should have absolutely nothing to do with the raw vegan movement. Anyone who takes any of these and claims to be hundred percent raw is basically kidding themselves. Heat processed foods are not raw regardless of temperatures used to heat them and any food that needs first to be processed should never be considered as ideal, least of all glorified with the title of "superfood"!

> Life can change for the better, just as easily as it can change for the worse.

Raw veganism is about eating one's food as nature offers it, if nature doesn't offer it as edible, nor as easily obtainable, you can be sure nature never intended for us to eat it; especially not in great quantities.

Supplements

I know there are people who swear by them, who insist that the earth has been depleted of nutrients and that this is reflected in the foods it produces, which they believe to be equally deficient. I do not share this belief. I believe that the real essence of what ails us, lies not in deficiency, but in toxaemia and that pretty much all dis-ease, no matter which cleverly coined Latin name it has been allocated, has the same basic cause. It is really quite simple; toxaemia. the gradual (or more rapid) poisoning of the body through eating, inhaling or injecting things which one basically shouldn't. Whether it be an outright poison, car exhaust fumes, heroin, petrol, cigarette smoke, alcohol, Mctucky fried pizza bagel pasta pies, coffee, or even plain old mashed potatoes. All will eventually pollute the body enough to cause it dis-ease of some form or another.

I may be wrong, but I suspect that the taking of supplements does no great favour to anyone. I'm more inclined to believe that through taking them habitually, one's constitution becomes lazy, slowly lessening the ability to absorb nutrients through natural foods. In some ways, not too dissimilar to how enemas make the bowels lazy! Perhaps as a last resort, or dire straights measure, supplements may serve some purpose, but as a general daily addition to one's diet, when eating otherwise correctly, I would not personally sanction their consumption.

I also understand that any scientific research conducted, biased or not, is based on a test subset of people that are all latently sick (they are all at varying levels of toxicity due to their flawed foods), thus test results and statistics cannot yield truly accurate informative results.

Other Raw Regimes

Raw veganism is not the sole form of raw diet being practised, far from it, there are people out there experimenting with all manner of raw diets.

Instinctivorism[64]

Tradition is no excuse for cruelty.

Originating from France, there is a group of people practising raw food eating, their movement is called "Instinctivorism". The followers call themselves Instinctivores, or "Instinctos" for short. As well as all the stuff you'd expect to find on their tables, they habitually eat raw, sliced animals too. The flesh is not just raw, but also left to lie around fermenting for a few days before consumption. Their theory and reasoning is that primitive humans were never themselves hunters, but belonged primarily to the collection of species classified as scavengers.

Carnivorous animals they basically divide into three distinct groups. Those that hunt and kill, those that hang around and wait for the killers to have their fill, so's they can move in and feast on the leftovers. Lacking the correct appendages, this is where we all supposedly fit in. The last lot are the rodents and worms and maggots that eventually help to clean the carcass from sight. Now, I'm not going to argue one way or the other about how humans may or may not have eaten in the distant past. I guess I would not be beyond persuasion to take a time machine and journey back to see us in daily action, but I'm not holding my breath waiting for the patent. And personally, I also admit very openly to extreme scepticism concerning the whole Darwinian evolution theory.

But, even if I were convinced that we did once upon a time hang around with grumbling tummies, waiting for the wolves to finish their dinners first, it still would make no difference to how I feel today. No theory will persuade me to feast upon the flesh of others as the Instinctos habitually do. No one will convince me that I must eat another, or die prematurely of malnutrition. I know that this is not the way the universe runs. Eating flesh is the grossest of all diets. The universe is built on love. Love is what makes it all go around. Even the most cold-blooded, murdersome individuals would not survive in their present corporal forms without love. Love is

"The basic foundation of humanity is compassion and love. This is why, if even a few individuals simply try to create mental peace and happiness within themselves, and act responsibly and kind-heartedly towards others, they will have a positive influence in their community." - Dalai Lama the driving force. Taking the life of another, and feasting on his flesh, is, the greatest of atrocities, totally out of sync with our true essence, which is nothing short of Divine hugfilled loveliness.

To give them credit, the Instinctos are generally of above average health, but this does not in the least surprise me, as the average is far lower than it could or should (or will) be. And to give even more credit, the main principle on how they eat has been a major inspiration for me and helped refine my diet to its current transitory form.

Generally speaking, they let their noses have first choice. Whatever on their raw tables smells most appealing is given highest priority to the mouth. They will eat a particular food, whether it be oranges, carrots, durian, dead sentient being flesh, birds eggs or plates of wriggling insects, and they will continue feeding on that one particular foodstuff until the body, through subtle messages, indicates that it has eaten enough. This may be signalled by a slight tingling on the lips or tongue, a change in taste, or another message from deeper within the body. This they call *l'arrêt instinctif.*

> You can't fix your health, until you fix your diet.

The instinctive stop

Once the *instinctive stop* has been reached, they will push their food aside and if they still feel their appetites have not been satiated, they will return to their tables, once more smell each item and choose the one with the most appealing odour. The pattern will continue, such that one meal may consist of two or three different types of food, until their hungers are satiated. Although I can't say that this is how I too choose my meals, I can see the underlying sense in doing so.

Instinctive eating only works provided your choice is of foods in their *natural* states. As said, the Instinctos eat wriggling maggots, live insects, rotting fleshful morsels, fish in decomposition and birds eggs, and consider it important that these be included regularly whenever the nose doth choose. Their philosophy does not accept milk, nor any dairy stuff to be valid table options, as these were clearly, to them, never a part of our original diet. It's a very well structured method of eating, but lacks compassion as it's based on how one man (Guy-Claude Burger[65]) believed primitive man once ate and lived (their philosophy covers more than diet alone) and does not take the rights of animals into consideration.

It is also a very social method of eating as it cannot generally be practised fully by lone individuals as very few of us have the economic wealth enough to load our tables with broad ranges of foodstuffs for each meal.

Instinctive eating can only be practised with a valid selection of foodstuffs. Given also the choice of mixed conglomerations, combination abominations and cooked monstrosities, the nose will generally lie to one's body about what it needs. These types of smell were generally never around at the dawn of time, so the human body does not know how to analyse correctly their value as food.

Our sense of smell is a highly powerful organ rarely given its full credit, and my overall feeling is that there is much to be learnt from the Instinctos, but that they themselves have a lot to learn about the true nature of life.

"If you don't like seeing pictures of violence towards animals being posted, you need to help stop the violence, not the pictures." - Johnny Depp

Paleo / Primal

Similarly to Instinctivorism, the Paleo Diet[66] and Primal Blueprint[67], are based on so called evolutionary science; the theory of how primitive humans once ate and attempt to guide followers to adopt the patterns of pre-agricultural ancestors. The two diets are often confused, as they have many aspects in common, but the basic difference is that the Primal Blueprint diet allows dairy whereas Paleo doesn't. I mention them both in passing, but as neither have a true understanding for the Golden Rule (explained in more detail in the chapter on religion), similar to the shod omnivores, they regard their food purely as food and disregard any sentience or objection the being it came from would have had in being chosen as a meal. I will not spend more time on them.

801010

The 801010ers[68] (pronounced eighty, ten, ten (ers)) are a more recent group of almost raw dietary vegans. The movement was founded by a guy named Doug Graham who also authored the book "The 80/10/10 diet[69]". Many of the 801010 crowd falsely refer to themselves as fruitarian, I intend to go into more detail with this in the next chapter.

Although not all of those claiming to adhere to this regime are themselves vegan, 801010 is also referred to as a LFRV diet (Low Fat Raw Vegan). The meaning of the numbers is a basic calorie guideline, where it is recommended that 80% of one's calories comes from carbohydrates, 10% from protein and the final 10% from fat and that those calories should come from raw fruit, vegetables, nuts and seeds.

There is no doubt in my mind that this conception has been of great assistance to many, encouraging and helping them to improve both their diet and lifestyle, however, for my own personal taste, I find that as well as grossly lacking in simplicity, (despite frequent claims made to the contrary by core members of the group), its focus is predominantly concerning health and fitness, thus lacks the crucial empathy component of veganism itself.

As I've stated in my introduction, I have no formal education, and to me all this talk of calories is just meaningless hot air. As a fruitarian, I also have no desire to even look at my food as a bunch of calories or carbohydrates, proteins and fats. I wouldn't recognise a protein under a microscope, and carbohydrates don't sound like anything I'm seriously ever going to need. Referring to fruit in such terms removes their beauty. Effectively semantically sullying and insulting them.

But hey, that's just me, and I guess whatever floats your boat or turns you on.

They often talk of fruit as fats and sugars too, which I also find degrading, and although I've always been somewhat mathematically minded, I still find all that counting

> Don't have an 'in your face' attitude about being vegetarian, vegan, raw or fruitarian. But don't hide the fact either. Be proud, yet humble. Be the best example you are able.

that they do, confusing. I think they have a sort of minimum guideline for the amount of calories one should eat daily, three thousand, and are always talking of carbing up and high carbs. They most definitely encourage over eating, recommending that when you are full, you force yourself to eat just a tad more, just to be sure, and consequently discourage one to trust in the bodies own innate wisdom to chose what it needs *given a valid selection of foods*.

I state that they are "almost" raw as some include cooked rice, and most if not all include nuts, seeds and dried fruit, (more on this soon) and I make the distinction that they are <u>dietary</u> vegan as the 801010 focus is predominantly on fitness and health, and thus there are clearly no guidelines discouraging leather belts, trips to zoos and circuses with animals, keeping pets or vivisectionally enhanced cosmetics, or even using nonvegan based B12 supplements.

Which brings us to the next flavour of raw thinking and the crux of this book: Eden Fruitarianism.

Every person you meet,
everything you hear,
every book you read,
every sight you see,
everything you experience,
happens for a reason.
What you choose to learn from them, is up to you.

"I don't believe in killing whatever the reason!"
- John Lennon

Most people sit on the back's of beings,
choking them, and exploiting them,
and yet assure themselves and others,
that they are very sorry for them,
and wish to ease their lot in any possible way;
except by leaving them alone,
and stopping doing what they are doing.

"You shall know the truth,
and the truth shall make you mad."
- Aldous Huxley

EDEN FRUITARIANISM

I began the previous chapter by telling you how raw veganism can also very much be an ethical choice. That is, *besides* the very valid moral duty we have to keep our own bodies healthy. Both Raw Veganism and Fruitarianism are missing crucial ingredients if they do not also focus on widening one's powers of empathy, ergo compassion and kindness.

I intend to lemon and limelight these issues throughout this chapter.

I believe it of utmost importance that the moral guidelines and health aspects, outlined in previous chapters be fully understood before one can be ready to succeed with Eden Fruitarianism, so if you have impatiently skipped forward to this chapter, I can tell you now you are missing out on the solid foundations around which this philosophy is constructed. If you haven't already done so, please take the time to read the previous chapters before continuing.

You say you love the world,
but you help in its destruction.
You say you love the sun,
yet you sit in the shade.
You say love the ocean,
yet you sully it with your toxic chemical sun-creams.
You say you love fresh air,
but you happily pollute it with perfume and cigarettes.
You say you love children,
Yet you feed them foods that make them ill,
You say you love cows,
but you stake and steak them.
You say you love lambs,
but you chop them.
You say you love fish,
but you bate, batter and butter them.
You say you love birds,
yet you cage them in and steal their eggs.
You say you love animals,
but what's that I see on your plate?
You say you love trees,
but you fell them.
You say you love flowers,
but you pick them.
You say you love carrots,
yet you uproot them.
You say you love the wind.
but still you close the door.
is it any wonder,
that I sit here confused,
when you tell me,
'it's love that makes the world go round.'
Now I am afraid also,
that you will say.
"I love you"

Fruitarianism

Firstly, there are probably as many flavours of fruitarians as there are of vegetarians.

We get vegetarians who eat everything but red meat, and others who eat chicken and fish, and of course the vast majority take dairy products and eggs. And yet the word itself sounds like it would depict someone that just ate from the vegetable kingdom. Far from it. Language is often illogical.

Similarly, we get fruitarians who eat roots, leaves, tubers, seeds, grains. Indeed, even whole plants. Shucks, there are people calling themselves fruitarian who cook or otherwise abuse their foods before ingesting and even those who are not totally opposed to eating the occasional morsel of flesh!

As a little anecdote, I recall some years ago a couple of friends of mine who went to meet a self proclaimed fruitarian living in Ireland. They found her at home eating

"Whatever we plant in our subconscious mind and nourish with repetition and emotion will one day become reality." - Earl Nightingale

bread with peanut butter and jam. In her mind, her meal was made entirely from fruit and seeds/grains which she supposed to be a regular part of a fruitarian diet!

There are fruitarians that mix it all together in astronomical, gastronomical onslaughts, and others that try to simplify by eating mono and some calling themselves fruitarian who will even try to convince us that it's dangerous to eat just fruit!

I suppose it is just the way of the world, and that all teachings are eventually perverted, distorted, warped and diversified. I feel quite sure (admittedly, perhaps naïvely so) that original vegetarians just partook of vegetable foods and never dreamed of supplementing their diets with milk from other species or birds eggs. Certainly they would never have considered themselves vegetarian, if they chewed and swallowed fishes or birds.

But language adapts itself and people who weren't vegetarian, became vegetarian, not by changing their diet, but just by the constant redefining of the word vegetarian until they became socially and linguistically accepted as being vegetarians, even though they clearly once wouldn't have been.

Thus out of necessity, new words spring into existence to help define where one really, dietistically and ethically speaking, stands. The word *vegan* is a good example, popping into existence in the 1940s, to describe someone who was *really* vegetarian. and later still the terms lacto-vegetarian, ovo-vegetarian, pesco-vegetarian, lactov-ovo vegetarian, even semi-vegetarian and socio-vegetarian became somewhat commonplace descriptive tags.

I fear that much the same has already happened to the term fruitarian. With people claiming that if 80% of one's diet is fruit, then one is fruitarian. This random percentage has been played with extensively, to allow more and more people to consider themselves fruitarian. 75%, 70%, 60% fruit. Make up your own percentage and become a fruitarian! Then I've seen people calling themselves lacto-fruitarians, which a couple of Swedish contacts I had in the past believed to be a sound version of fruitarianism; which involves capturing, imprisoning and stealing the milk of other species. Of course there are all the 801010 fruitarians too, notorious for telling people that 100% raw, fresh fruit is not only infeasible, but also dangerous and many of whom still haven't fully grasped veganism, let alone raw veganism.

Looking at the word fruitarian, you would think that it means someone that just eats fruit. Agreed, that seems logical enough, but the truth is that the very vast majority of people out there labelling themselves as fruitarians, do make exceptions to the "just fruit" rule, most of them on a regular daily basis.

With this in mind, I'm going to be brave and coin a new term. *Eden Fruitarianism.*

Teaching a child not to pick flowers, is as important to the flowers as it is to the child.

Defining Eden Fruitarianism

Eden Fruitarianism is, I believe, the original fruitarianism as practised by the once-upon-a-time couple of Adam and Eve. It can only be reached through a full understanding of the aforementioned "isms" (so get back there and read them if you haven't already!) and is predominantly a philosophy based on ethics, requiring the very deep realisation and understanding that of all the food available in this world, the only nutritional substance which is truly given, and thus has the potential to be totally free of any violence, is FRUIT!.

Plants make use of a variety of ingenious methods to disperse their seed[70]. These methods include taking advantage of gravity, wind, the flow of water and the movement of animals (where the seed hooks itself onto the fur of a passing animal). Some plants are even able to make use of ballistic/mechanical dispersal, where a seed pod explodes, outwardly flinging its seeds away from the mother plant[71]. Probably the most successful technique many plants employ, is to encapsulate their seeds in an often vibrantly coloured, fragrantly odorous, deliciously tasting flesh that many animals, including humans, naturally find appealing. This is one of nature's ways to give the seed a chance to be moved some distance away from the mother plant.

Clearly, in such cases, the plant wants other life forms to consume this fruit flesh.

Bacon would not be a choice if the pig had any say in the matter. A lamb, given the gift of speech, would most probably say "no" if you asked if you could eat her leg. Fish would no doubt choose to stay in the water, if they could and I feel pretty sure turkeys must object once their Christmas fête (or should that be *fate*?) is made clear to them. Chickens are surely protesting from having their eggs systematically stolen and freedoms restricted, and both cows and their calves would be up in arms, if they had any, with the theft of their milk and violent separation. Given the chance, bees will attack and defend ferociously, even sacrificing themselves in the process, in order to protect their precious honey; a sure sign they do not part with it voluntarily.

But even for the things which have no oral or physical ways to defend themselves, it does not take a great leap in thought and faith to understand that they too, given the ability to do so, would likely protest.

Eating a carrot involves destruction of the whole plant, the lives of lettuces and cabbages are brought short once picked. Even individual leaves torn off a plant, seem in some way to me, to be against the grain of a universe I believe to be built on love. Eating grains, cereal, nuts and seeds generally involves depriving those capsules of any real chance of a life that could have been theirs.

What is Beethoven's favourite fruit? Ba-Na-Na-Naaaa!

Plant Perception

If you believe that such plant life, lacking an obvious animal comparable nervous system, cannot feel pain and you are unable thus to feel empathy for such life forms, I might suggest you read The Secret Life of Plants[72]. It should offer some insight into generally unseen plant life communication and emotional expression.

Published in the first half of the 1970s, the book details experiments conducted on plants that were hooked up to a polygraph; a basic lie detector of the era. The results proved beyond reasonable doubt that plants would react and respond to violence toward themselves as well as surrounding plants and animals. Indeed, not only do they react to such negative stimuli, but even to the mere *threat* of such action! Experiments showed it was enough to even think about harming a plant for it to react; to scream out in protest. Screams that rarely get heard and recognised. If this seems a little far fetched to you, then please take the time to watch this short video[73] from the MythBusters[74] team who basically were able to confirm the findings of the 1970 scientists. If after watching it, you are psyched to see more, try this short (under three minutes) youtube video[75]. Or if you feel up to it, watch the full length youtube documentary[76] (just over one and a half hours) of the secret life of plants.

Also, more recently, the university of Aberdeen conducted a study[77] that showed how plants communicate amongst themselves, warning each other of approaching pests and threats. Fascinating reading.

By showing this, I am not trying to say that taking the life of a plant equates to taking the life of an animal. It should be clear that even though a fruitarian acknowledges the consciousness of a plant, and attempts whenever possible to minimise harm to any, we are likely all able to weed or end the life of unwanted plants, despite that recognition. Faced with the choice of taking a knife to the throat of a calf, or pulling up a carrot, no fruitarian will wonder which option is worse. Of course, if fruit is available, then such choices need not be faced at all.

> Honour life in any shape or form.

The Uniqueness of Fruit

Move on to fruit and you'll notice that it is a whole different kettle of fish. Or should I say *basket of mangoes*!

Going once more back to the 1970s, toward the end of the decade this time, back in the days when I used to work on giant computers in large false-floored, air-conditioned rooms, I got hooked on a computer game. probably the very first dungeons and dragons game ever written. It was a single user game called "adventure", or "advent" for short. Basically involving a labyrinth of rooms and corridors, with a surprise around each corner. One of the creatures one regularly encountered in that maze of twisty little passages all alike, was a troll. The trolls were unique in that the only food they ate was coal. Back then, I used to think that all food was taken against the best wishes of whatever life it came from, and that the world we lived in was unavoidably cruel. The trolls I thought had evolved something wonderful. They just ate coal and in theory were able to live totally at peace with their surroundings.

Of course, eating coal was never something I seriously aspired to doing, but I couldn't help but wonder how the world might be if all we needed to eat were raw, inorganic materials found in abundance everywhere.

Do something today that your future self will thank you for.

It took me years to recognise fruit for its comparable potential. Contrarily to other foods, given the gift of a set of vocal cords, the plant that bears the fruit, would most likely be singing "Eat them! Eat them! Here they are!". Because through eating the fruit, one will be helping the tree spread its kernels. And the more tasty the fruit, the more likely one will be to nurture and care for its seed.

To my knowledge, short of becoming breatharian, fruit is the only viable, usable solution to the *live and let die* scenario we currently find ourselves ensnared within. I repeat myself: Fruit is the only food that is genuinely given, thus karmically free and thus *the* only food (discounting inorganic materials, such as coal of course) that is truly compatible with a universe whose fundamental principal and driving force is one of love.

With this in mind, Eden Fruitarianism involves eating or genuinely aspiring to eat a diet consisting of 100% raw, fresh fruit. I probably still need to clarify the term fruit though, as there is clearly confusion among many as to exactly what a fruit is. I have for instance seen reports online of people saying things like "I eat 100% fruit" and then, going on to more closely describe their diet, will list that they eat greens, nuts and seeds too.

"If you love a flower, don't pick it. Because if you pick it, it dies and it ceases to be what you love. So if you love a flower, let it be. Love is not about possession. Love is about appreciation." - Osho

Defining Fruit

When I talk of fruit, I am referring to the often edible part of the plant that surrounds the seed of the plant. Durian, mango, nectarine, chocolate pudding fruit, chempadek, apples, oranges, strawberries, bananas, pineapples, cherries and other such obvious fruits are just a few of the countless species of fruit that spring immediately to mind.

Despite not always being classified as fruit, the following also belong to that category: Avocado, tomatoes, cucumber, zucchini, peppers, pumpkin and even eggplant and belladonna (deadly night shade). Clearly, the flesh surrounding the seed is not always edible by humans, thus there are many types of fruit that are not suitable food for us bipeds.

In some cases, such as the banana and the pineapple, the seed is often no longer present, these are however still types of fruit. Although rare in the western world, varieties of both still do exist however containing seed.

In other cases, such as the tomato, the kiwi, the pomegranate, the passion fruit and the strawberry, to name but a few, the seed and the edible flesh are basically inseparable, thus eating the seed too is unavoidable. However, in such cases, the seed generally stands to profit from the experience as the digestive process will help kick start whatever enzymes are in the seed needed to get it germinating. Thus the deal is symbiotic for both us and the plant. Provided of course we are not just flushing our waste down the WC!

What's Not Fruit?

Homer: *Doughnut?*
Lisa: *No thanks, you have any fruit?*
Homer: *This has purple stuff inside, purple's a fruit.*

Well. Obviously not meat, fish and eggs, nor cheesy yoghurty slime. Not roots, nor leaves, nor tubers, nor nuts, nor legumes, nor grains. Even if raw and even though some do consider these to be regular parts of the fruitarian diet, they ultimately do not form part of an Eden Fruitarian's fare. We see beyond things as been merely food or not and empathises with the history of our meals.

Difference Between Fruit and Nuts

I keep seeing people writing that botanically speaking, fruit, nuts and seeds are the same thing. I can sort of understand where they are coming from, by some definitions, everything that comes from the flower, is considered in some way to be the fruit of a plant. However, from an Eden Fruitarian's perspective, although they are clearly in physical proximity, they are no more similar than a root and a leaf. Playing with words suchly, a calf could equally be said to be the fruit of a cow and one's baby the fruit of one's womb, or even sea food being called Fruit of the sea. Clearly atrocities are committed when any of these are eaten.

Think of a nectarine, what we eat is the precious, sweet, nectar flesh that surrounds the stone/seed of the plant. The seed is clearly separate from the flesh. The flesh is the thing that is, so to say, given karmically freely. Think of a melon, what we eat is the deliciously tasting flesh of the melon. Not the seeds in the centre which generally get left out of the digestive experience. (Yes, I'm aware that some cultures roast them, but fresh out of the fruit they are none too appealing in my eyes). Think of a papaya, we eat the life giving, juicy, vibrantly colourful, sweet flesh of the papaya. the small black seeds get released back into nature. Or should. Think of an apple. The flesh is savoured, the core, discarded. I could continue ad infinitum.

Clearly not every seed is surrounded by this, so clearly precious substance, called fruit. Some seeds/nuts/grains etc. are void of the encapsulating fruit flesh. That's just the way the world is. *Not every plant consists of a fruit*. Not every plant consists of a seed either, for that matter. Nature is abundant with variations.

> "Life is an echo, what you send out comes back. What you sow, you reap. What you give, you get. What you see in others, exists in you. Remember, life is an echo, it always gets back to you. So give goodness."
> - Chinese Proverb

So What's Wrong With Nuts?

Well, that's a loaded question. I'm not trying to say here that anything is *wrong* with nuts, but then again, I'm not saying anything is wrong with seeds, grains, shoots, leaves, roots, tubers, insects, fish, mammals or other animals. Although there might be - ☺ .

However, I just don't believe any of the above are ideal foods for humans.

But about nuts specifically. Besides clearly not being fruit, I think it's well worth acknowledging, that unlike fruit, *commercially purchasable, **raw** nuts are simply not available*! I've had people write to me and say, *but David Wolf is selling raw almonds or cashews* etc! Don't be fooled. It's simply not true. If it is, then it's because he means something else by the word raw, than I do right now.

When I say raw, I'm talking of unprocessed raw. About raw, ripe and fresh. When others say they are selling raw nuts, then what they are most likely selling are processed (sun or air)dried nuts, about as raw as their shrivelled goji berries.

As described in the previous chapter, all natural, fresh, ripe and ready foods, eaten mono on an empty stomach, have what the French have christened an "instinctive stop". *Dehydrated foods, including nuts, have **no instinctive stop***. At best, they're physiologically a second class food. Your body will crave the addictiveness of them, thus be unable to truthfully tell you that enough is enough.

As an experiment, I'd like you to go out in nature and find some truly fresh (I.e., not even sun dried!) nuts and sit and eat them. I think you will have had enough of them far sooner than you ever would with those readily picked, de-shelled and packed store bought ones.

Truly fresh nuts, are slightly wet and soft. Not dried and crispy/crunchy!

Thus an Eden Fruitarian avoids such dehydrated foods, favouring also grapes over raisins, plums over prunes and fresh mango over dried, withered, dehydrated mango. To summarise, I avoid nuts for the following reasons:

> Sam: *You don't like raisins?*
> Joon: *Not really.*
> Sam: *Why?*
> Joon: *They used to be fat and juicy and now they're twisted. They had their lives stolen. Well, they taste sweet, but really they're just humiliated grapes. I can't say I am a big supporter of the raisin council.*
> Sam: *Did you see those, those raisins on TV? The ones that sing and dance and stuff?*
> Joon: *They scare me.*
> Sam: *Yeah me too.*
> - Benny and Joon

1. Ethically, I'd like to give them the chance to fulfil their potential treeful destiny.
2. They are commercially not available raw.
3. I don't consider them to be physiologically ideal foods. Too heavy.

What About Coconuts?

Well, yes, granted, unlike other nuts, they are definitely readily available, raw ripe and fresh and in abundance for some. Physiologically, I'd reckon for that reason alone they'd have to be better for us than most any other nut available. However, they are still not fruit!

I love to see coconuts fall down when they are ready, and sprout in the sand. Coconut palms are a beautiful sight. And I have personally made the choice to try

> " Every time you are tempted to react in the same old way, ask if you want to be a prisoner of the past, or a pioneer of the present." - Deepak Chopra

and avoid ending the life of another prematurely. Of course, that's my choice and I respect that others may not feel the same way. We all have to reach our own conclusions about such matters.

I understand when people tell me there are an abundance of nuts and that by eating some, we may also help propagate others. Yes, if that's how you feel about them then great, enjoy them! My belief, which I'm not claiming is infallible, is that fruit offers superior nutritional benefits and is ultimately the least harmful choice. Thus I'm choosing, to stick to just fruit.

I think another thing we might observe about nuts, is how difficult they are to get in to. Think about it, every fruit, when it's ready, will grant you easy access to the flesh. Try and get into a coconut with your bare hands, or a macadamia nut with your teeth and that's a whole different story. Without a tool of some kind you stand little chance of getting at the edible interior.

In addition, although the husks may make good mulching material, the shells of coconuts take significant time to break down, and if not disposed of sensibly, all it takes is a quick downpour for them to become perfect breeding ground for mosquitoes to thrive in!

What About Legumes, Peas and Beans etc?

I see. Well, you can certainly get them fresh and ripe to eat, that's for sure. But I still don't consider them as fruit. Botanically or otherwise. They are seed and to be honest, although I've made occasional exceptions in the past, I'd rather let the seed be.

> "The Garden of Eden still exists; there are just no people in it." - Marty Rubin

I'm choosing to be fruitarian, because I believe it is the garden of Eden diet and because I'm a hopeless romantic that believes it's love that ultimately makes the world go round, that "love is all you need" and that fruit is the only food that fully has the potential to be compatible with that notion, being not only the highest of all foods (physically and spiritually). but also the only food that is truly symbiotically shared by any living thing.

There are however a couple of exceptions with legumes, that make certain varieties suitable fare for the Eden Fruitarian. Carob and ice cream bean (inga bean) are two such exceptions, where either the pod itself, or in the case of ice-cream bean the fluffy packaging encompassing the seed is both desirable and edible and serves the same purpose as the flesh surrounding other seeds. That of encouraging the eater to carry away the seed from the mother plant and distribute it further afield.

Mushrooms

Suffice to say mushrooms are not fruit and thus not the idealist of foods, however, as foods go, they are far from being the worst choice one can make. I have little really to say about them, but I think for all such similar questions, it might be wise to refer to the section coming shortly called "The Ethical Food Tower".

Nutritional Science

Off the Cuff

The only solution -
Stop the pollution!

I'm allergic to calories. They make me sweat and fart and froth and burp. Carbohydrates are killing me slowly, when I look at photos from thirty years ago, I can see how much they've aged me. Vitamins have played their role too, with some hair loss and not to mention the minerals that have destroyed my teeth. And then there's those dreaded glycogens, proteins and polypeptides. Who knows what havoc they've inflicted upon my body over the years!

Oh how I wish I had grown up in a world full of fruit and with guardians with sense enough to understand its life giving properties. I could have avoided all those ghastly amino acids and sugars that have (rav)aged my body.

My simple understanding of a calorie, is that it's a unit equal to the amount of heat required to raise the temperature of one gram of water by one degree at one atmosphere pressure, and as such I fail to see what business they have playing vital roles in our diets. The mere thought of them sets my spine a shivering. It's rather like eating empty hot air, don't you think?

In my opinion, all that pseudo science, of microscopically dissecting the molecules of our food before eating them distances us from the pure simplicity of eating the fresh, juicy, ambrosial, heavenly

100

scrumptiousness of fruit. It degrades the sweet and saporous, dribbilicious nectarine to a mound of health threatening sugars and other pathogens. The durian gets transformed from a delectable hunk of tantalisingly custard, creamy, peerless, spiritedly irreproachable bliss, into a congress of lifeless decaying vitamins, ugly nefarious fats (god forbid!) and gremlinous amino acids.

Thus we have the meat and dairy industry that cleverly marketed us the protein myth, the raw fooders who sell us their goji berries with all their magical built in ingredients, and now the new set of fruitarians who insist that we need to understand microscopic food content before we can hope to do it properly. They want for us to believe that we cannot do it ourselves, but need expert opinion and guidance to get there.

Take a simple apple and cut it in half. After barely ten minutes what do you observe? The two halves exposed to the air, are likely already beginning to discolour. Slowly becoming increasingly more brown. Put very simply (because, let's face it, I ain't no scientist!), what's happening is the life force of the food is slowly dissipating. The longer you leave it, the less value it will have as a food.

Now, take another apple and grate it. You'll observe that the smaller the pieces, the quicker they'll discolour (oxidise). i.e., the quicker the true value of the food is lost. If you start doing stuff like subjecting the morsels to heat or similar, then the process is yet more rapid and far more devastating!.

> Eden Fruitarianism is the solution to the dilemma of the *screaming carrot.*

In order to observe those pesky impalpable little vitamins and their ilk, food has to be dissected so small that by the time it's sandwiched between the glass under the microscope, you can be sure that any vital, once present, life force is long gone.

Same goes for the amino acids, glycogens, carbos and the ever elusive calorie? I mean, yeah sure, you might text book quote me any of it, but admit it, really you're just blahing stuff that you have no idea about. How many of us would even recognise a plate full of pure B12 if we saw it? And yet so many tend to talk about them, feigning a familiarity that is nothing short of fictitious.

I don't care for any of it. I also don't believe that anyone can rightly say what anyone else should specifically eat at any given meal. If you think that you need someone to guide or tell you, then you surely haven't understood the simplicity of true fruitarianism. I don't care if someone tells me I ate just forty calories yesterday, or four thousand, to me it means nothing, so I'm not into calorie restriction, nor the opposite of force feeding myself, nor castigating anyone else into believing they need to get a certain amount each day. I don't give a damn how many grams of food I ate in my last meal, and I'm not into ritually forcing drink down my gullet to stay hydrated in the future.

The next time someone comes up to you and tries to get you to eat protein or calories, be strong, say "no thank you" and turn and walk the other way. Resist the temptation, eat fruit, live long(haired) and prosper.

> "Only until all of mankind lives in harmony with nature can we truly decree ourselves to be an intelligent species."- Genelle Haldane

Seriously Though

Okay, tongue out of cheek, it hasn't always been the case that I've avoided nutritional science. Way back, when I first became vegetarian, I was slightly obsessed with the subject, reading up on it through whatever books were out there at the time, determined to succeed with vegetarianism, followed very soon thereafter by veganism and believing that only through a sound knowledge of science would that be possible. Once upon a time, for example, I knew the name of every single essential amino acid the human body was said to require and not only their complex individual names, but also their general function and in what vegan foods they could generally be sourced. Nowadays, I can't even recall if there are supposed to be eight, nine, or ten essential amino acids and don't remember the name, or particular function of any one of them.

> "I do not like eating meat because I have seen lambs and pigs killed. I saw and felt their pain. They felt the approaching death. I could not bear it. I cried like a child. I ran up a hill and could not breathe. I felt that I was choking. I felt the death of the lamb." - Vaslav Nijinsky

At some point along my path, I reached an epiphany, realising that if every major change I had made to my diet was indeed an improvement, which I solemnly professed to believing, then why was I suddenly obsessed with the possibility of nutritionally failing? Surely if each step was truly an improvement, then I should have been less and less concerned about each individual microscopic element of nutrition. After all, most people go through their lifetimes without ever thinking about vitamin A and iron and there I was fretting over whether or not I was getting adequate amounts of both, even though, I profess, I had no real idea what either of them were. It was like a part of me didn't have faith in the path I'd taken, most likely because the vast bulk of the rest of society was in opposition to what I was feeling, believing and practising and because at the time, I lacked confidence facing that opposition.

The more I delved into nutritional science though, the more I noticed that there were an awful lot of conflicting ideas being peddled, which basically meant that at the end of the day, it was up to me as an individual to decide which of the many and varied, opposing viewpoints I believed in, with no way to certify that any were genuinely correct, even though all were somehow purportedly based on supposed proven unshakable scientific fact. Thus, not having any real idea what a complex carbohydrate was, nor how to verify if what I was reading about them were correct, then at the end of the day, it was still all about belief and trust that someone else genuinely knew what they were talking about.

It became clear to me too, that whenever any nutritional science research is funded and undertaken, it is pretty much always done so with some kind of ulterior motive. Probably the bulk of money spent on nutritional research has been funded as part of some kind of marketing ploy, and as such, results sometimes achieved through methods that one might describe as mendacious, or more charitably, *less than honourable*. Research says that we need protein for healthy cell growth and tissue maintenance and meat contains protein, ipso facto we encourage you to eat meat. No one seems to question how the beef got so full of protein eating just grass!

> The sooner we wake up and realise that we have a moral duty to guide and protect this planet, the sooner things will improve for every form of life on this planet.

We need calcium for healthy bones and teeth, and milk is an excellent source of calcium. In today's world it's not always easy to get as much iron as we need, therefore we propose you buy our unique brand of iron tablets. See how this kind of research can and has been, on countless occasions, used in advertising. Just because it's written down somewhere, just because it's a shared common belief, doesn't make it fact! And even if someone has purportedly scientifically proven something, this does not mean that YOU "know" it to be true too. The most you can say is that you trust that everyone else knows what they are talking about.

Protein

In fact, we have all been constantly fed such biased conclusions, that we often go around quoting them as gospel. This is the main reason people are always asking vegans where they get there protein. The question itself implies that the questioner really has an understanding of protein, something which is very rarely even remotely true. If I picture chewing on one, it is bland, dry and like chewing an old boot. I don't know what they look like, and neither do I care. Sure, I understand them to be purportedly made up of amino acids, and before the body can assimilate them, they must first be broken down once more into those self same acids. But one has to see how distant a protein is from the reality of food. If you are walking through a garden, and find a cherry tree, sit under it and enjoy the small, purple, bliss bombs until satiated, then lie down to rest on the grass, smelling the sweet wafting fragrance of flowers, and listening to the melodious song of birds, the last thing on your mind will be "I wonder if I got my full complement of proteins?

It appears to be the case that *not getting enough* protein is a lot more difficult than one might expect and to succeed in protein deficiency almost requires one to be starving oneself. It is said for example, that roughly 0.9% of human mother's milk is protein[78]; and this being nature's intended sole food for a human, at probably the most rapid growth stage of our lives!

> "The secret of change is to focus all your energy, not on fighting the old, but on building the new." - Socrates

This would seem to imply that such small percentages of protein should generally be easily adequate throughout other stages of one's life too. As it happens, the protein content of a broad range of fruit is said to vary from between roughly 0.5% to 3%, which should be far more than adequate to meet one's supposed needs.

Not yet convinced. You might be surprised to know there are even raw food body builders out there[79], that manage to bulk up despite obvious meat deficiencies. I read this morning that a group of fifteen vegans competed against hundreds of body-builders with traditional omnivorous, heavy meat, dairy, and egg based diets. The results: The vegans won five out of seven divisions that they were in[80].

But, it isn't my intention to delve further into such questions. If it interests you, you might check out The China Study[81]. Research that I'm told proves the superiority of a vegan diet! I also recommend Ross Horne's book *The Health revolution*[82] which delves more deeply into the science behind a fruit centred diet.. I am quite certain that if examined unbiasedly and truthfully, science has the potential to one day prove beyond a shred of doubt that a hundred percent raw, fresh, ripe fruit diet is superior to all other diets, but even should such a theoretical day come to pass, it is likely that some will choose to not believe its credibility. Instead they'll choose to keep their faith where their ingrained habits already lie. Again; in the end it is all up to us as individuals to decide what we believe to be true and what not.

Even if we were to self experiment with every conceivable diet, it can sometimes take years for consequential health problems to become apparent. Get a well read vegan and an equally well read Paleo guy in the same room, and both will swear blind that research has proven undoubtedly that their own particular individual diet is nutritionally superior. From a purely nutritional outlook, they could argue ad infinitum and get no where.

Faith

That's why I don't desire to go there. Eden Fruitarianism is not about nutrition, or any

> "Fear is the path to the dark side, fear leads to anger, anger leads to hate.. hate leads to suffering" - Yoda

accompanying set of pseudo science "facts", it is about ethics and ultimately faith that there are ethically correct alternatives that are to the benefit of *all* sentience involved. Thus, whether we are willing to accept this or not, any nutritional choice relies on faith of some kind. Most people are not (willing), they mistakenly believe that they have knowledge and indefatigable science to back them up, but all they really have is faith that their information source is reliable, and that results have been interpreted correctly.

I am personally choosing to forsake nutritional science entirely and place instead my faith with the concept of *live and let live* which I believe to be a valid path. This does not mean that you too should do so. By all means do whatever research you feel is necessary. Other than vague warnings that an all fruit diet may be lacking in something, there seems to be nothing more specific than that. Not enough minerals, some will say, but push them to find out what specific minerals and no one can tell you. Mostly they are all quoting each other, and truly valid non-biased research has yet to be properly undertaken.

To me, it makes a kind of intrinsic sense that whatever is truly best for the environment, will also be best for us as individuals. Whatever is best for the ecology, will be best for the long term health of whichever economy is employed. Whatever is best for our health must also be the best for the health of the planet as a whole and all sentience involved. That the path of do-as-little-harm-as-possible, will not only be the most beneficial for all those we come in contact with, but also for those following that path.

"When man learns to respect even the smallest being of Creation, whether animal or vegetable, nobody has to teach him to love his fellow man. Compassion for animals is intimately connected with goodness of character and it may be confidently asserted that he who is cruel to animals cannot be a good man." - Albert Schweitzer

I believe that the currently popularly shared belief of *live and let die*, that in order to live, someone or something must die, is inherently flawed and serves no real use other than to help keep the world ensnared in its dark ages. I believe that Eden Fruitarianism offers a long term solution to this dilemma, it nurtures empathy and although I cannot truthfully entirely and clearly envision where widespread adoption of the philosophy will lead, I have every faith that it is into the light!

This "faith" in doing the right thing for all parties present and concerned, is of utmost importance in succeeding with Eden Fruitarianism. Without it, one cannot truthfully claim to be on its path. One must have an understanding that surrendering to this path, will likely cause an onslaught of opposition and one must be prepared to face that opposition calmly, peacefully and with full faith that whatever obstacles are strewn in one's path, however thick and irksome they may seem, there is always a route through them, however troublesome the obstruction, it will always ultimately be surmountable. And remember, the great white spirit never gives us more than we are capable of handling!

"The difference between stumbling blocks and stepping stones is how you use them." - Unknown

Such obstacles will come in the form of seemingly overwhelming opposition from apparently well meaning kith and kin, your own nagging doubts about whether Eden Fruitarianism is anything more than the crazy thoughts of an insane minority, or an onslaught of health issues all connected to the fact that your body is finally cleaning itself. It is understandable that without an underlying strong faith that what you are doing is of undeniable benefit, failure will be predictable. Remember at this stage, you are a pioneer; not every one is pioneer material.

Naturally I have my own experiences of that which I talk. The onslaught of opposition from friends etc. The ridicule and accusations of extremism. The temptations and struggles and many stumbles. The accompanying ongoing detox. All, or any of this, is enough for many to forsake the path and to return to the familiarity, comfort and security of the sheeple flock. I think the occasional stumble is inevitable and don't see stumbling, in and of itself, as a problem. The importance with Eden Fruitarianism is keeping the faith. Lack of faith and the accompanying fear that one is failing have already deterred many. Such challenges await us all.

"The only people mad at you for speaking the truth, are those who are living a lie." - Unknown

As an example, a few years back (while on a hundred percent fruit diet). I went through a period of experiencing extreme fatigue. It was literally the case that I could barely walk a hundred meters without feeling exhausted and having to sit down, or rest. This went on for an uncomfortably long period of time. I could have consulted a doctor, who would no doubt have informed me I was suffering from low blood pressure and prescribed drugs to raise it, or (if they had even bothered to enquire) drawn the conclusion that my diet was surely to blame, but I didn't. It's likely low blood pressure was indeed a symptom, but as I could see no reason why I should be suffering from such, other than detox, I decided to wait it out. Sure enough, about one year later my energy levels returned to normal, without having done anything but persisted on my pursuance of Eden Fruitarianism!

No one cares about your protein intake, until they find out you're vegan.

I also understand that any scientific research conducted, biased or not, is based on a test subset of people who are all latently sick (they are all at varying levels of toxicity due to their flawed foods), thus test results and statistics cannot yield truly healthy informative results.

The way I see it, there is one major cause to what ails us, with many varying symptoms. The only real lasting solution; stop the pollution!

I think humans have barely scraped the surface in regards to our limited knowledge of how the body functions and all it requires to do

107

so. As an example, I used to know this guy who had been diagnosed iron deficient, and this despite that he was eating proliferous amounts of animal flesh (doctors orders!). Similarly, there are a great deal of flesh eaters out there who still find it necessary to supplement their diet with vitamin B12. Considering that meat is purported to easily contain sufficient quantities of both iron and B12, it seems odd that their needs are not being covered by their diet. Such cases confirm my suspicion that deficiency itself is not the real issue, but rather lack of ability to absorb, through physiological contamination from poor food choices.

Biological Transmutation

In cases where it has been supposedly proven that certain nutrients are lacking, biological transmutation steps in as one theoretical way of explaining how our needs for a particular nutrient may be met despite its apparent absence in one's diet. It posits that if a physiological body is healthy and free of toxins, that it has the ability to basically transmute certain elements already in abundance within the body into the ones it requires.

> By eating flesh, one eats murder. By doing so one expresses indifference and ignorance, not love. Every meal is a major expressions of our love for the world.

For many, this will indeed sound like a pseudo-science and indeed it may well be, I'm not claiming it as fact, although there is ample evidence out there which seems to indicate it may be. If you've never heard of it before, I suggest you google it and you will see there are many people who take it quite seriously.

Like I've said, I'm no scientist and as stated I neither personally need, nor necessarily trust the validity of supposed scientific explanations currently available. For my own needs, I simply don't really care for any of it.

> If you don't believe in miracles, perhaps you have forgotten that you are one.

Vitamin Tablets

By this point, it should stand to reason that I see no value in vitamin tablets. If I look at them, all I see is dead inorganic matter that I seriously doubt can do anything to genuinely help anyone. Whenever a new element is recognised and isolated, you will find some company somewhere that will take advantage of this fact and begin selling said element through clever marketing. "Yes, science has proven that you need phytosyllium for shiny thick hair ma'am" "I guess I'd better get some of that then". Such an ad is guaranteed to work especially well with those who, due to warped food choices, have dry thin dull and brittle hair!

Sugar Issues

I find it somewhat distressing that so many people refer to fruit as "sugar". The 801010ers are particularly fond of this, proving their ignorance to the role of fruit, yet still calling themselves fruitarian. Sugar has a bad reputation and rightly so, it's a highly refined fully denatured product obtained through processing the hell out of sugar cane or sugar beets or similar. Then there's fully natural, designed by nature for us to enjoy and thrive on, fruit. Whatever is inside fruit, bears no kinship with sugar[83]. Sure, from a denatured scientific viewpoint, it may contain fruit sugar, "fructose" as one of its constituent elements, but while that fructose is still locked intact and an intricate natural constituent within the fruit, it has none of the detrimental effects associated with sugar. Use a chemical lab to separate the fructose though, and its value will decrease to the magnitude of the synthesised vitamin B tablets. So if you are one of the many that confusingly refer to fruit as "high in sugar" you need to seriously consider changing your vocabulary. Personally I think I'd prefer to call fruit sugars, fruit sweetness and avoid the sugar thing altogether.

Diabetes

So even if all the doctors in the world (which thankfully is not the case!) were to advise a diabetic against taking too much fruit, I would adamantly and rebelliously keep my stance and disagree with them all. If anything, it is precisely due to the lack of fruit (and consequent increase of overly cooked foods, especially meat and wheat) in their diet that they may have diabetes in the first place!

"Society has always had its visionaries who talked of love, beauty and peace. - But somehow the "practical" men have always been there to praise the smog as a sign of progress, to preach *just* wars, to restrict love while giving reign to hate. It must be one of the greatest ironies of history, that today the only solutions for the "practical" men, lie in what they think of as the dreams of the idealists. The question now is; Can the realists be persuaded to face reality in time?" - Paul Erlich

Hey, I warned you I don't do science! Don't take my word for anything. Naturally distrust me. That's what I want to instil in people. A natural distrust in authority and the written word. Just because a doctor (or anyone) says something's true, doesn't make it so. Just because something is written down, that doesn't make it true. And like I said, I've no formal education. I just see things from a different vantage point and I can't make you see what I see. I cannot give you my clarity. All I can do is describe to you what I see.

Suffering from any flavour of disorder does not pre-empt/exclude one from embracing the Eden Fruitarian lifestyle. Nothing does. Not one's age, certainly not one's gender nor race, not even one's state of health. It's a philosophy meant for the entire world. No exceptions. And its practice is nothing less than uncle Tom's miracle cure all.

Teeth

I've heard it said by many that adopting a fruit based diet will cause unavoidable damage to one's

> Go on, cross the bridge, then burn it!

teeth. Indeed I myself have lost several teeth over the last couple of decades and I can understand how some people fear that a fruit or fruit centred diet may be responsible for that and internal nagging doubts, remind them of all the scaremongering about too much fruit sugar and the effect it may have on one's teeth, bones etc.

The truth behind my own tooth saga will be fully documented in my autobiography, but cutting a long story short, it was not due to eating solely fruit. My own teeth problems began way back as a shod omnivore. In my early twenties it became an almost normal occurrence that at each of my six monthly dentist visits, I pretty much inevitably ended up having at least one filling. One particular check-up saw my dentist tell me I was in need of ten fillings. nine normal ones and one root canal filling. I had my teeth built up on several occasions, partially for cosmetic reasons.

> "You don't need treatment. The fever, inflammation, coughing, etc., constitute the healing process. Just get out of their way and permit them to complete their work. Don't try to 'aid' nature. She doesn't need your puny aid - she only asks that you cease interfering."
> - Dr. Herbert M. Shelton

Fast forward to my path to fruitarianism and I had long abandoned all desire to regularly have my teeth checked. Over time, the work done on my teeth began reaching its sell by date, which mixed with my own struggles with cooked food addiction, and through eating too much unripe fruit (which I cannot emphasis enough, being not yet ready to eat will have its consequences, and likely none too pleasant ones!), my teeth slowly fell apart. For sure, had I been stronger willed, more determined, I could have avoided that issue altogether. But I wasn't and I learned my lesson the hard way.

It would have been great if I'd succeeded in reaching fruitarianism without any dental damage, I would have been able to proudly show off my full set and say, "look! a fruit diet is fine". But for me, part of my journey took me through that hardship and despite a year or more of on and off excruciating agony (probably some of the worst pains I've ever experienced, to the point of delirium), I managed to avoid ever consulting a dentist.

"There has to be a revolution. But it has to be a revolution of consciousness. A spiritual revolution!" - Russell Brand

This I did despite an enormous amount of peer pressure that bad gum infections could potentially lead to brain damage and death, I knew that I was on the right path and that eventually, I would pull through. Which naturally, I did.

Yes, it's true, I have the same aversion toward dentists, as I do towards doctors, they are both part of an industry that has no real benefit from us being healthy and will offer no lasting assistance toward that goal[84].

Like the GPs who on the pretext of supposedly helping us, deal out their symptom suppressing drugs (for which, similar to the street drug dealers they are greatly financially rewarded), the dentists, short of advising us to not eat too many sweets and to brush our teeth regularly, offer us no real knowledge as to why our teeth might not be perfect. This is most likely because the industry as a whole is ignorant of the role that diet plays in our healths, including the effect the standard overcooked "flesh and two veggies" diet will have on our teeth.

The "medical industry" is one of the world's largest money spinners and would have to seriously restructure and minimise itself, should we all turn around and eat what we were supposed to eat.

Why did the tomato go out with a prune? - It couldn't find a date!

What makes me so sure that it wasn't just eating predominantly fruit that caused my teeth to fall out? Well, that's easy.

1. Since getting through that period of time with very weak teeth, my teeth have, if anything at all, strengthened themselves within my mouth (clearly, had the issue been fruit alone, my teeth would have progressively deteriorated and would still be an issue and causing me problems, which they are not, despite all those nasty beastly fruit sugars and the increasingly less frequent brushing).

2. My teeth were already in a very weak state prior to my unripe mango adventure, their health having been compromised on my previous cooked food diet, and the ever present assistance from what I once believed to be well meaning dentists, who had already given me a mouthful of countless fillings.

Of course, the fillings are still an issue, as since adopting my philosophy of non interference and letting my body heal itself, some are still intact. And occasionally, one might reach its use by date and disintegrate or fall out, but I don't mind. I am glad to see the back of them! I've been told I should have them removed, as they mostly all contain mercury and there is the issue of poisoning, but I am sticking to my non-interference method and intend for things to go their natural course. Besides, I feel such an invasive procedure as mercury filling removal, may do more harm than good.

Also, I believe that the body if left to use its own inner wisdom, may possibly grow a third set of teeth; there are documented cases, although rare. If this should happen, all well and good, if not, no worries. I'm not holding my breath.

Apart from the cosmetic issue of missing a few teeth, I really don't make a big deal of it and the remaining teeth I have do their job in regards to chewing my food.

> "Most of our so-called thinking processes are devoted to finding excuses for going on believing as we already do." - Dr. Herbert M. Shelton

Different Body Types

Back in the 1990s, while living at El-Faitg, in the French vegetarian/vegan community of Douceur et Harmonie, up in the mountains close to the Spanish border. There was this elderly woman there, the founder of the community, her name was Viviane. If she's still in the same body today, then she would surely by now be pushing 100. Viviane had this theory that we all have different physiological/nutritional needs and that some of us are just unable to live well on an all raw vegan diet, let alone on solely fruit.

I recall she wrote about it in a small quarterly newsletter she edited and published at the time, making a comparison to how the horse chestnut tree and the sweet chestnut tree, although looking similar, had very different needs as far as their soil was concerned; one preferring it more acidic, or something similar. She said the same was true for humans, in that we may all look similar, but our nutritional needs were actually different.

At first glance one can be forgiven for following her line of thinking, but her logic was clearly fundamentally flawed and as much as she may have been right that horse chestnuts and sweet chestnuts looked similar, they were nevertheless two completely separate species. Like she was comparing Pandas to Polar bears. Had she compared sweet chestnut tree, to sweet chestnut tree, she would have seen that they all had the same basic requirements.

Similarly (sort of), ancient ayurvedic philosophy, divided humans up into three main body types (or doshas as I believe they called them)[85], each with different nutritional requirements (pitta, vatta and kapha). The more modern version, especially since the advent of the book Eat Right For Your Type[86], divides people up depending on their blood type. The theory goes that people with "Type A" blood are best off as vegetarians, while people with "Type O" blood are natural born zombie flesh eaters. "Type B's" are somewhere in the middle, needing cheesy yogurt lasagnas no doubt.

But I propose that they are all wrong. We are far more similar than any of these philosophies care to admit. Other mammal species also have different blood types, and yet no one would try and tell you that certain dogs should eat certain foods, and others a quite different diet, or that some cows should eat grass, but that others would be better off eating predominantly alfalfa! Of course at any given point in time, our individual requirements may differ, but overall we are all fundamentally physiologically alike. Our stomachs and hearts are generally in the same places, as are our kidneys, liver and lungs, all serving the same anatomical purposes.

They told me I had blood type A, but it was a Type-O.

What the proponents of "diet types" are seeing, is apparently different types of people. But these apparent different types, are just different bodies having been consistently abused in different ways.

Once the body returns to a truly good state of health, it will become clear how those seeming differences were nothing more than self inflicted, and that we are truly all fruitarian. Nothing will sustain us, maintain us, nurture us and help us evolve as a species more than returning to a fruit centered diet.

The Ethical Food Tower

We've all seen the "Food Pyramid" chart, on a classroom wall, or in a doctor's waiting room. It's one I believe to be fundamentally flawed, as it promotes foods none of us should be eating. I propose therefore a new concept. An ethical food tower.

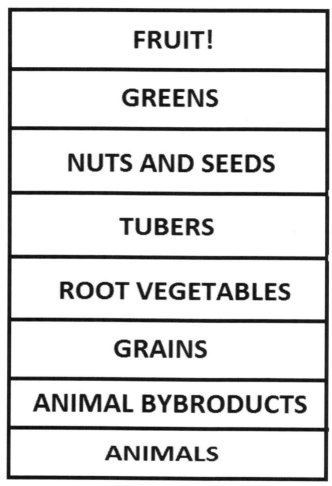

ETHICAL FOOD TOWER

Unlike the traditional food pyramid we are likely all familiar with[87], the tower differs in that only purely raw ingredients are listed. Thus you'll note the obvious absence of foods such as breads, cakes, pizzas, chocolate and ice-cream. Other than that, although visually there are some similarities between this tower and the many varieties of the traditional food pyramids in existence, the predominant difference lies not in the contents, but in *how the tower should be read and interpreted.*

Designed by the US Department of Agriculture and dating back to the 1960s and '70s, the basic principle of the food pyramid is that we eat predominantly from the lower rank and proportionally balanced from the others. The overriding focus of this new proposed chart is one of ethics. Instead of offering a guideline, or rough percentage, of what foods one should eat, it shows the order of crassness of the foods, with the lower ranks being more Neanderthal in nature, embraced more by the dark side, and the summit being fruit, the highest of all foods, and the food we should all aspire to be eating. The goal is to eat as high in the tower as possible! The tower supposes that all this food be eaten in a hundred percent raw (ripe when appropriate) natural state. Once the cooking process is included, things get much more complicated, and additional layering would be called for, with a great deal more potential for overlap. The tower looks roughly like the diagram on the following page.

You will note, that the bottom layer contains the edible(?) flesh portions of animals, every mammal, fowl and fish you can name etc. Slightly above it, with some overlap not made visible, (I'm no artist), I stick the so called by-products of the animal flesh trade, and other items that originate from deliberate animal abuse, i.e., dairy and eggs. The overlap is diffuse and not altogether clear. The next layer up, are the grains, which due to their environmentally destructive monocrop origins, and need for heavy post harvest processing should never be considered as ideal foods. Move up a layer again and you'll see the root vegetables, the carrots, parsnips and turnips etc. things that necessitate the direct, unavoidable and intentional killing of plants.

Above that, but again with a slight overlap (depending on production methods), the tubers, like potatoes, yams, sweet potatoes and Jerusalem artichokes, things which on a small scale can potentially be harvested gently from the ground with minimal harm to the plant, and if care taken the food can be eaten and eyes cut out from the potato or similar to regrow new plants.

At any given moment, you have the power to say "This is not how it is going to end!"

Moving up the tower one more notch, once more with the ever potential for overlap, I would place nuts and seeds, but think they should only ever be eaten if truly fresh, thus with the instinctive stop still intact. Anyhow, above the nuts, I'd place greens, again, there is definitely room for overlap, as methods of growing and harvesting surely play a role, as with small scale home gardening, many greens can be harvested in a far less destructive manner than traditional farming methods allow.

Then, right at the top, is the fruit.

Truth be known, the tower is far from finalised. Clearly I've missed out some of what gets eaten, like crustaceans, snails, frogs, insects, grubs and the like, which I'd probably place in that vague area between layers one and two and three, then there's seaweed, algae and mushrooms which I suppose should be toward the top end of the tower somewhere. Further precision could be made within each layer too, with for example tree fruits being higher than the likes of tomatoes and cucumbers and then there are other factors like the proximity of the food and transport issues which may mean rearranging things a little.

For simplification lets say the interpretation of the tower is suited purely for foods that are all 100% organic and locally grown.

Clearly, if there is no fruit around and one must eat other things, then move down a floor or more,

"If you want to awaken all of humanity, then awaken all of yourself, if you want to eliminate the suffering in the world, then eliminate all that is dark and negative in yourself. Truly, the greatest gift you have to give is that of your own self-transformation." - Lao Tzu

as far as you feel comfortable, with the understanding that the bottom layers are really *no go* zones. Of course, the ultimate goal is for us to settle in environments where the foods we are comfortable with, are readily and affordably available, or to bring that environment unto us.

It should be abundantly clear from the layers, that I am not equating the uprooting of a carrot to the murder of a lamb and if you wish to, you can add a bottom layer to the pyramid with humans too. The cutlets shanks, chops and flesh for the cannibals amongst us. In doing so, it can then also be abundantly clear, that I am not fully equating the murder of an animal, with the murder of a human. This should appease all those that might think I am putting the welfare of animals above that of humans. I think undermining either is an abomination!

Why did the tomato blush? Because it saw the salad, dressing.

If you can cut out the bottom layers, including the grain, then you are already making fine progress. Let your spirit rise upward with your meals.

Mono Eating

I should make it clear to begin with here that although many of our meals are basically mono we do also regularly mix some fruit together and although I can see there are clear benefits to eating mono, in the grand scheme of Eden Fruitarianism, I don't tend to place a great deal of emphasis on doing so. If you're eating up there on the top of the food tower, and have an understanding of the basic concepts outlined within this book (there's more controversy to come, so hold onto your hat and finish reading before you nod your head in agreement!), then congrats to that!

The reason for this lack of emphasis is that Eden Fruitarianism, as I've already clearly stated, is NOT a diet but an ethical choice and once you see that and have moved up into the top of floor of the tower, it is a matter of personal choice as to whether or not you refine your diet yet further. (a personal growth choice that Eden Fruitarianism heartily encourages!).

If mono calls out to you, I can see there are advantages of eating that way at times. Especially it should make clear the superiority of fruit above other food. Try flaying the skin

"4.6 billion years old, scaling to 46 years, humans have been here for 4 hours, the industrial revolution began 1 minute ago. In that time, we've destroyed more than half the world's forests." - Greenpeace

from a cow and biting in to her, now try peeling a mango and sampling that. Which do you prefer? Try getting on your back under a lactating goat and drink directly from her udder, and then try picking some fresh strawberries and eating them. Then compare the two experiences. Chew your way through a plate of raw wheat, and then one of fresh grapes. Face a bowl of diced carrots, and then an equal amount of cherries. Which of these choices offers the most pleasurable experience? A plate of dandelion leaves or a plate of durian?

My belief is that by unbiasedly facing our foods in this way, it will eventually always be clear that fruit is more colourful, more flavourful and overall more enjoyable an experience.

Because shod omnivorism has lost sight of this mono simplicity (which clearly has its merits), you'll often find people eating a complexing amount of foods simultaneously, confusing and overtaxing the digestive system, thus slowing it down unduly and rendering the body unnecessarily sluggish.

If we (Květa and I) mix fruit together, we tend not to get any more complex than tomatoes, cucumbers and avocado as our often regular afternoon meal. Sometimes there might be zucchini in there too, or capsicum, but rarely anything more complex than that.

Fruit's Not what it Once Was

People find many objections to eating fruit, one common one I hear is how fruit has been changed so much over time that it is no longer as it should be, that it is often mineral deficient or has absorbed excessive amounts of chemical pollutants through the air.

I don't think anyone can deny that all the above may at times be true, however the one thing one should see is that of all the foods available, *none of them* are quite as they should be. These issues and similar can be addressed toward any of Earth's food. If you think that fruit is sullied and that pig flesh isn't, you are deceiving yourself.

Despite imperfections, fruit is still a clear, best choice for all involved. It is our duty to recognise that, and to do our utmost to help restore the planet to its potential splendour, gradually healing the soil to once more be healthy and rich, for its fruit to be purified.

I often think this whole "demineralised fruit" issue is mostly scaremongering. If it is true, I have not noticed the effects of that demineralisation and although any of the undesired chemicals that happen to be present are surely not ideal, fruit contains enough cleansing properties of its own, to help ensure they don't linger too long within the body, but are pushed through with the normal physiological cleansing process.

> How is holy water made? - Boil the hell out of it!

Water

There exists a popular thought. It's been around for several generations and like many thoughts that have been around a while, often gets quoted as fact. Many claim that the human body needs to drink eight to ten glasses of water a day in order to maintain one's health. Where this idea originated is not something any nutritionist can answer, even the ones who will insist it's correct!

Of course, I don't think anyone will claim it's a hard and fast rule, more like a basic rule of thumb guideline, based upon a variety of factors such as size, gender, age, physical condition, climate, activity level and, most importantly, diet!

So although there may be some truth to it, in that an average person of average gender, age and health and on an average diet, may require something approximating eight glasses of water daily, the same can certainly not said to be true for someone on a truly raw or Eden Fruitarian diet!

By its very nature, the Eden Fruitarian diet is high in fluid, with many of the fruits eaten, containing 70%, 80%, 90% or more liquid, reducing one's need for water to a bare minimum. Indeed most days I have no need at all for water, I would be over exaggerating if I said I drank an average of six litres a year. Květa does not drink any.

Although a basic guideline for water intake may likely serve its purpose for those on more conventional diets, where the high water content of most real foods eaten is generally systematically removed first through the heat process, the idea of taking a certain arbitrary quantity of water on an otherwise hundred percent raw vegan diet (i.e., no nuts and dried fruit too!) seems rather foolish to me. Rather like the idea of taking in a certain amount of calories daily. I think once one understands what the real food intended for us is, and makes positive steps to return to such a regime, we will all begin once more to trust the body's inbuilt wisdom. Listen to it and it will tell you if you are genuinely thirsty or hungry or not. You don't need to pay a so called diet guru to tell you what and when to eat and drink, you just need to understand what constitutes as a real food!

> "I never drink water because of the disgusting things that fish do in it." - W.C. Fields

Children

One should not think it is necessary to wait until adulthood before embarking on the Eden Fruitarian path. Its benefits can be reaped regardless of age. There is no better choice we can make for our children than to begin them along its path. The longer we wait to do so, the more arduous it will be to reach that path. Don't take my word for it, if you are not convinced, go ask your GP!

Seriously though, my belief is that Eden Fruitarianism is a path suitable for everyone, not only suitable, but ultimately yearned for by the universe and that as such, we are never too young, nor too old, to begin upon it. From the vantage point of the path, all it takes is observation of small, shod, omnivore children to understand this. How quickly they are able to get sick and detox. And how quickly they can recover! This will likely seem paradoxical, but their quick to sickness

119

is a sure sign of their little bodies being healthy and vibrant. We may ignorantly lament over their suffering and blame other parents and children for passing on their bugs and sniffles, all the time being oblivious to the underlying fact that it is really us that is jeopardising their healths through encouraging them to eat unsound food choices.

Persevere on the shod omnivore path and at a certain point our children will appear healthier and no longer constantly struggling, fending off childhood bugs. This has nothing to do with them being healthier though, but more to do with the body gradually resigning to its often lost cause of struggling against foods it was never designed to process. Of course, with our bulging waste lines and warped senses of what constitutes good food, we are rarely able to recognise any of this.

If we are fortunate enough to understand this, we are then faced with the issue of guiding our children back on the right path. This will not be straight forward. One can rightly expect protest, complaint and outright tantrums. One has to understand they are coming off a drug and as such, they will experience symptoms of "cold turkey". Be there for them. With sound help, guidance and above all patience and understanding, they can get through it.

> "Children who are spanked are more likely to exhibit depression, anxiety, drug use and aggression as they get older. The more they are hit, the more likely they are to hit others, including peers and siblings. As adults, they are more likely to hit their spouses. The secret is that spanking not only doesn't work, it is totally unnecessary. When children are raised with age-appropriate expectations and limits accompanied by empathy, they tend to behave and cooperate. So if you were spanked and think you came out alright, it wasn't because of the spanking. You'd be even better if you hadn't been spanked!" - Dr. Laura Markham

Even if you, as a parent, still struggle with the addiction of cooked and overly processed non-foods, once you have understood the detrimental nature of such foods, it will be your moral obligation to not let your children follow the same health destructive path. Think of it as if you are a smoker, struggling to quit. If you yourself can't find the strength and commitment to break free of the habit, would you think it acceptable to let your child smoke too? I am not suggesting you forget your own struggle, because unless you too can follow your convictions, there is little chance that your child's success will be lasting.

Environmental Issues

It is a sad fact, that this planet we call home, has been and continues to be violently trashed. The predominance of that trashing has been through the hands, thoughts and deeds of our very own species. Guilty as charged. Our consumer habits necessitate exploitation, whether it be of slave labour, the innocent imprisonment (and ultimate bloody slaughter) of other sentient species, the widespread destruction of arable land and forest, pollution of air, water ways and oceans and ultimately our own individual healths. Of course, none of this is necessarily immediately apparent, but pretty much everything purchased in any mainstream outlet store has its impact.

For many years deforestation has been ongoing at an ever more alarming rate. By some reports, as much as, or more than seventy percent of the world's forest areas have been flattened within the past two hundred years, much of that within the past few decades. It's as if the planet is now forced to breathe with less than one decrepit lung!

> Those who believe they have no time for healthy eating will sooner or later have to find time for illness.

At first glance one might think with the overwhelming negativity of it all, that there is no escaping any of it. Indeed, short of totally going bush and growing one's own fruit food through completely sustainable methods, it is currently virtually impossible to avoid some contribution of negative impact.

An individual stepping onto the path of Eden Fruitarianism should not expect to see immediate global changes, that would be just unrealistic, and much as many might judge the idea of Eden Fruitarianism to itself be unrealistic, I believe there is a profound realism that supports it. One should not be overly concerned with what everyone else is doing, but focus purely on lessening one's own carbon footprint. As a consequence of fully embracing Eden Fruitarianism, suddenly many of one's once popular consumer items will no longer be of appeal and thus, by the very nature of things, our impact will lessen. I am not talking purely of food here, but of pretty much everything else on the supermarket shelves which isn't in the fresh produce section. No more cans, no more excessively packaged cereals, no more cleansing products, no more oils, no more conditioners, no more denatured junk foods. The list is longer than most pieces of string.

Indeed, it is safe to say that most commercial businesses will ultimately reach their demise once Eden Fruitarianism has been fully understood and adopted by the majority. This is a good thing!

Agriculture

I wish to make clear once more, that similar to veganism, Eden Fruitarianism, is not a diet as such. This is what distinguishes it from other flavours of fruitarianism. Unlike the traditional omnivorous or vegan diets that are based primarily on annual crops, predominantly cereals, a fruit based diet is predominantly based on perennial agriculture, primarily fruit tree growing. As Eden Fruitarian consumers, we will be demanding more fruit, more trees will need to be grown.

Being reliant on annual crops means heavy reliance on fossil fuels for land cultivation. It involves wide spread loss of wildlife habitat and annual unintentional slaughter of innocent animals that get caught up in the heavy brutal machinery used to turn the earth. The earth suffers from this practice, which is, to say the least, highly unnatural. For ethical vegans this should be reason enough to at least forsake the third floor of the Ethical Food Tower!

In nature one cannot find a naturally grown field full of *one* particular plant species. Mono crops are devastating the planet. To grow large mono crops to feed the masses, involves a constant struggle against diversity of plant life. The alternative of not relying heavily on pesticides, herbicides and other chemicals, is even more labour intensive, resulting also in higher produce prices.

> What's the difference between boogers and broccoli? - Kids don't eat broccoli.

Fruit tree growing does not involve the earth being disrupted each year, by heavy rotavating ploughs and the like. Which is not saying fossil fuels and chemicals are not used in fruit production, far from it. The amount and impact is however vastly reduced. And I mean **vastly**. Fruit trees are currently also grown in large mono orchards. Field after field of mango etc. And ultimately I clearly believe this can also be improved, however the environmental consequences are far less than the desertification tactics of annual monocrops.

It takes up to fifty thousand litres of water to produce one kilogram of beef compared to only two and a half thousand litres to produce one kilogram of rice and **significantly** less still for tree based agriculture producing one kilogram of fruit[88].

Land Animal Farming

The UN have released a report titled "Livestock's Long Shadow[89]". They explain how the animal exploitation industry, major suppliers of unhealthy addictive foods, are one of the *most significant contributors to the most serious environmental problems the earth is currently faced with.*

The solution? Move away from animal farming and mono cereal crops and begin focusing more on horticulture and small diverse fruit tree orchards. Not only will this help restore the planet to its one time splendour, but ultimately save and prolong lives and serve to awaken awarenesses.

> *The line of gooselings, follow their mother. Their tiny webbed feet, slap the muddy path*
> **- Allan Hart.**

In addition, animal industries habitually negatively impact biodiversity through causing loss of native habitat, introducing non-native species which leads once again to unnecessary competition for both food and water[90].

The solution is clear again, to use land to plant more trees, creating more biodiversity and offering a long term solution to food production through environmentally sustainable fruit growing techniques.

Additional detrimental impacts animal raising has on fresh water supplies (all of which can ultimately be avoided by ditching dark aged flesh eating habits), are that livestock often trample and destroy river edges and pollute water ways. Native vegetation is systematically destroyed to make way for monocrops or pasture land which will ultimately cause soil erosion and effect rainfall[91].

The manufacturing of leather and other so called animal by-products is a major source of pollution, with its reliance on formaldehyde and other toxic chemical pollutants[92].

In the US, animal factory farming pollutes more waterways than all other industries combined[93].

A large chunk of greenhouse gas emissions can be attributed to conventional animal farming techniques. Take into account the fuel and energy consumption such farming methods rely on and the statistics are surely even more disturbing. Animals raised for food in

Australia alone produce about 3.1 megatonnes of methane annually[94]. (Methane has a far greater global warming potential than carbon dioxide).

Believe it or not, grazing takes up nearly 50% of the Australian continents arable land. Roughly 380 million hectares[94]!

Instead, we could be planting more intermixed varieties of fruit trees. Eating more fruit and ultimately cutting the meat, wheat and cheesy dairy from our diets, is a very effective way for individuals to make a very real difference to reducing global warming.

Additionally, livestock animal grazing has a direct impact on the environment through compacting and acidifying soils, by increasing to unsustainable levels the volume of manure, and other by-products, effecting both land and waterways.

According to the CSIRO[95] and the University of Sydney a massive 92% of all land degradation in Australia is caused by animal industries.

Increased numbers of agricultural animals, over-farming and overgrazing has lead to vicious cycles of deforestation, erosion and habitat destruction. Eventually this will lead to starvation prompted by the disappearance of plant food sources.

> "Mindfulness can be summed up in two words - pay attention. Once you notice what you're doing - you have the power to change it." - Michelle Burford

Fish Farming

Meanwhile, out in the ocean, innocent fish are being caught by the tens of thousands, all to satisfy human gluttony for their zombie flesh eating habits. The consequences are that these modern fishing methods have depleted populations to such a level that the industry is now targeting deep sea fish, species not previously taken[96].

Not only are fish populations being forced into a spiralling decline, but destructive fishing techniques including dragnets, long lines, purse seine nets and drift nets are destroying large parts of the ocean environment in the process. By unintentionally capturing other sea animals such as non-target fish species, whales, dolphins, turtles, seals and sea birds like the albatross, many of these species are facing extinction due to fishing. Insatiable gluttony for food with eyes has created vast areas of the ocean void of desirable fish.

All this mindless destruction while the only real food that encourages a healthy body, mind and planet; fruit, goes virtually unrecognised for the solution it harbours.

Fish farming is equally insane, creating concentrated faecal contamination in specific areas of the ocean and rivers, promoting the rapid spread of disease and parasites, to both captive and wild fish populations. Even more bizarre is that farmed fish are even fed fish; between ten and twenty kilos of wild fish is needed to produce a kilo of farmed fish[97].

Crikey, that was one boring screed! I just wrote it down and read it back to myself and all I could hear was "Blah blah blah". In future do your own google research, won't you?

I could continue listing insanities, many of which, probably together with yet more mind-numbing ones, are available on the internet, but what would be the point?

The only real solution is very clear to me. Leave behind destructive habits reliant on the slaughter of fellow beings and their homes and instead plant fruit trees and eat their luscious offerings; the most superior of all nutrition and the only truly environmental friendly and truly karmically free food. FRUIT!

If you stick with fruit, only you can know what and how much appeals at any given point in time, don't ignorantly expect someone else to tell you what, when or how to eat; it is folly to believe that anyone knows better than you do.

How, When and What to Eat

The rules are so, so simple really. Once you've pushed through the fear and uncertainty, the only thing you really have to understand is the valuable role and potential of fruit to restore peace to the world. Once you have that, all you then have to do is present yourself with only fruit to eat and trust your own body to intrinsically know what it needs. Sit down, look at your food, smell it if you want, feel it, grok it. Hungry for a cucumber, then eat one. Feel like tomatoes. Eat as many as you want as often as you want, whenever you want. Still hungry but want something different and avocado looks appealing, then eat one or as many as you want. Feel like mixing them all together. Go for it!

Don't make the 801010 mistake of ruling avocados as fats. Avocados are a fruit. Lumping avocados in with nuts, is a flaw in their pseudo science. As stated, all commercially available nuts are cooked, thus their overall effect on the human physiology, is bound to be comparable to cooked food, and ultimately detrimental. Avocados are neither nuts nor cooked, nor heat treated so their effect is very different, and not comparable to that of nuts. Don't be afraid of them, be afraid of the pseudo-scientists who would rather blind you with their half-arsed science and bring you to a sense of fear that they alone have the complex knowledge you need to stay healthy.

Don't get caught up in calories, omegas, antioxidants, free radicals and electrolytes (things you will likely never really understand anyway!), or forcing yourself to eat more than you need. Become yourself a free radical. Don't get caught up in drinking copious amounts of water even though your body doesn't feel like it, just because some snake-oil salesman tells you you should. Stop looking for other people to tell you when and what to eat and just go with the flow and conviction that fruit is your food and it matters not about analysing which micro-elements are in each food, just trust your own physiological wisdom to guide you! If you feel like eating banana and tomato mashed together, then go for it!

Once I saw the world with open eyes, I realised I'd come here to change it.

Unless you are underweight, you'll not put on more, even if you eat fruit all day. If you are fat already, then you will lose weight until you reach your ideal one, which by society standards will be considered skinny, but only because society is fat. If you look at a fruitarian diet with the preconceived notion that you'll never be able to succeed with it, then you will be setting yourself up for failure. Seriously give it a shot and you may be surprised to discover just how little fruit is needed to keep one satiated and how a simple large glass of orange juice can give us enough energy to keep us going for longer than one might think.

Simple rules: Eat when hungry, drink when thirsty, rest when tired, sleep when sleepy, shit when... Shitty? (It's a known fact that being constipated can make one angry!). Don't eat and drink for tomorrow. You're not a camel living in a desert!

"Time to go run the calories away, do away with all the numbers stalking you, throw out the bad habits and excess weight." - Alysha Speer

To avoid issues of not getting enough, avoid situations where there isn't an easily accessible plethora of fruit. It's no good planning to do a bike ride or long walk and force eating and drinking everything you think you need before you start out.

Locally Grown Produce

It should be clear, that the closer your food is grown to where you live, the better it will be for everyone and everything involved. Currently there are all manner of procedures fruit and food in general, must endure before being transported vast distances. The least of which being the fuel used. Should the food cross national boundaries, far worse treatment often awaits it. Such treatment is known as phytosanitary measures[98], and frequently involves extended processing of the food even before it leaves the farm of origin. The supposed goal is to prevent importation of pests through food trade, and this will often involve irradiation, dipping the produce in an insecticidal soap or light paraffinic oils, and further treatment with fungicide (to control post harvest rot). As a rule, these are all processes NOT undergone when the food is grown and bought locally.

All the more reason why the committed Eden fruitarian should make sincere long term plans to relocate to where the fruit is grown!

A wife, being the romantic sort, sent her husband an SMS: "If you are sleeping, send me your dreams. If you are laughing, send me your smile. If you are eating, send me a bite. If you are drinking send me a sip. If you are crying, send me your tears. I love you!" The husband replied, "I am on the toilet. Please advise."

Shit Happens

Once we have had our meal, the inevitable happens. Nature calls. It is generally said that human waste is not a good addition to the garden, the main reasons you'll see quoted are health issues and there's often this feeling that it's much more dangerous to use human manure than any other animals' in your garden.

Well, I think this piece of folklore has been disproved in many places, as human sewage is sometimes treated and used as fertiliser on farms, but if there is a shred of truth to it, then the truth is centred around the stinking faeces of the cooked shod omnivore. The waste of a fruitarian is comparatively much cleaner and far less intensely smelling and thus more beneficial for the earth. Eden Fruitarianism recognises this and encourages us to stop flushing such waste to unknown fates with the sewage

"What's the difference between toilet paper and a shower curtain?" "Oh, so you 're the one!"

works and instead take responsibility for all our waste, recycling it as best we are able.

Consider also using water to clean your behind instead of toilet paper. After all, if you had shit on your face, you wouldn't just wipe it off with a tissue and think, "it's clean now".

> "Life is a tragedy of nutrition" - Arnold Ehret

Fitness and Exercise

Any quick google search will show that many of the batch of novo fruitarians out there have a strong fixation on some kind of fitness regime. This may be daily sessions at the gym, a strong desire to run fixed or variable distances daily, or some ingrained desire to forever push the limits of their bicycling endurance.

Such exercise is not altogether mutually exclusive with Eden Fruitarianism, but preoccupation with alpha egos, six packs, abs, biceps, triceps, steal buns, competitively outperforming one another and an often morbid fascination with apex predators and survival of the fittest, is completely absent and there is recognition that the best form of daily exercise has goals beyond pushing oneself to beat individual or group records.

Why run around the garden, expending energy solely for one's individual fitness, when one can be using that energy to dig holes to plant new trees, to climb trees and harvest their fruits, to weed and mulch around those trees, or to prune the dead branches from them?

Such actions can be both rewarding and meditative, use up just as many calories (whatever they are?) and far less likely to result in physical injury than the harsh running on concrete, the breathing of conditioned air in gyms, or the dodging of traffic on one's push bike.

Personally I don't see pushing oneself to the limit as being ultimately that beneficial and more likely to cause injury than more gentle techniques that can be employed like yoga, walking, swimming etc. (or, again, a healthy relationship with one's garden!).

Weight Loss and the Biggest Loser

> I keep trying to lose weight, but it keeps finding me!

Whether or not you are into daily exercise purely for the goal of personal fitness, weight loss is a virtual inevitability on the Eden diet. Weight loss has pretty much always more to do with diet than exercise. I'm not sure if you've ever seen that TV show "The Biggest Loser", Květa and I used to watch it some years ago, back when we still had a TV. The basic premise of the show is that they get a whole load of obese people, split them into two groups of a red team and a blue team and make them compete to lose weight, with one member being voted off from each team each week. They teach everyone to eat healthier than they were, while meanwhile turning them into trained athletes with rigorous daily exercise routines.

The Green Team

We used to talk of how it would be great to have a third team, the green team, that would be put on a cleansing fruit juice cure and an Eden Fruitarian diet. Instead of being taken through boot camp comparable training, they would be merely given gentle daily exercise routines, like swimming, walking, yoga and gardening. Not being pushed to the limit until throwing up, but just mild movement.

While the blue and red teams are being taught about calorie counting and good and bad cholesterols, the green team, under the shade of some large fruit tree, are being given lessons in empathy and compassion; the precise lack of which, being the real reason they find themselves in such awkward body predicaments!

THE INVISIBLE MAN LOVED MESSING WITH WONDER-WOMAN

Instead of being out in the hot sun, or in some air conditioned gym exercising relentlessly, we would take them on field trips, let them witness the birth of a calf, let them see how the mother gently cleans it afterwards and then let them see the agony of separation. How both the calf and mother suffer and call out for each other. Let them witness the conveyor belts of chicks waiting to be sexed and show the destiny of both genders. Teach them

129

about branding, tagging and debeaking. Let them see the factory farms and the lifelong incarcerated conditions of animals destined to be gluttonously feasted upon. Let them witness animals as they are prodded and shocked toward the delivery trucks where they often spend hours packed in overburdening conditions on their final arduous journeys to the slaughterhouse and let them see the slaughterhouses and hear the screams of animals defenceless to change their destinies.

Show them the same animal species in unfettered realms and teach them how each one is as individual as any cat or dog or you or I. Let them see how every living thing desires a life of freedom and relative comfort void of fear and threat. Take them to see monocrop farming and teach them how it's a constant struggle, an inevitable losing battle against nature. Let them really see what their dietary habits entail, so that they may later make more informed choices and live with clearer consciences and minds, with more bliss and less in ignorance.

> "As long as we remain, at core, a culture that sees animals merely as commodities and food, there is little help for our survival." - Will Tuttle

We'd tell them to take their shoes off and go for a walk in the grass. Take them to beautiful nature spots and let waterfalls massage them. Teach them that being fat is never ever due to genes nor water retention, nor being big boned, and that even glandular issues can be rectified and everyone who's overweight can and should lose weight. No exceptions!

Perhaps we're wrong, but Květa and I are both convinced that the green team could quite easily beat the blue and the red one each week. The pounds and kilos would literally melt off of the participants!

> Addiction brings apathy. Break the apathy, and you break the addiction.

Eden Fruitarianism Continued

This is not all there is to Eden Fruitarianism, there are more aspects that merit their own section and are thus discussed in the following chapters.

130

SECTION TWO

ADDITIONAL EDEN FRUITARIAN
LIFESTYLE CHOICES

"They who dream by day
are cognizant of many things
which escape those who
dream only by night."
-Edgar Allan Poe

BAREFOOTISM

Once Eden Fruitarianism is fully understood and embraced, shedding one's shoes is a natural consequence. I think we all secretly love the feel of freed feet, the flow of fresh air upon them and the unimpeded ability to wriggle one's toes, and at some point the desire to liberate one's feet supersedes any desire to conform to the dictates of fashion.

""Healthy feet can hear the very heart of Mother Earth." - Sitting Bull

After a while you may grow to consider shoes as perhaps the ugliest, clumpiest items of clothing humans regularly don. It has become a complete mystery to me, how people are so attracted and attached to them. Some to the extent of developing a complete shoe fetish, obsessed with forever widening their collection, with dedicated wardrobe space and a pair to match every outfit. I fully sympathise with the ancient Greeks, who, according to wikipedia[99], viewed footwear as self-indulgent, unaesthetic and unnecessary.

It should be clear that the wearing of footwear volitionally is an exclusively human characteristic. I can get the practicality of shoes worn under certain circumstances. During sports, like skiing or football, or in temperatures experienced during winter months, or hot hot sands in the heat of the summer, or the sharp rough rocky terrains of some areas in nature. But the more one habituates one's feet to the freedom of being barefoot, the more tough they become and the more they can handle such extreme circumstances.

"To be barefoot outside doesn't just involve your feet - the rest of you has to be outside too. You get to connect with Mother Nature all around. Feel the sunshine on your face; hear the wind in the trees. It's easier to connect to a higher power when you're in touch with Nature." - Unknown

It feels good, to have the earth between my toes and to no longer have my feet restricted to confined sweaty spaces. I no longer even own any footwear. I stopped habitually wearing them back in the early 1990s and have not worn any since boarding a plane back in 2006 and then only while walking through customs and onto the plane!

I read once that original Australian Aboriginal peoples, with their ever nomadic lifestyles, would habitually be barefoot, and were they to come across terrain too difficult to pass through comfortably, would sit down and make themselves footwear from woven reeds or grasses or tree bark etc. They would walk through the rough terrain and then discard them, letting nature once more claim them. I think they knew quite well, the importance of keeping contact with the earth through the soles of one's feet.

Nowadays shoes are fashioned from any manner of exploitive materials and through many a manner of exploitive methods. The most expensive from the flayed hides of butchered animals and also more commonly these days from destructive petrochemical by-products.

"Barefoot, is becoming a healthy hobbit"
- Yoda, Jedi Master

Confronted with the notion of not donning footwear, many may immediately prejudge the idea as dirty, unhygienic and a sign of poverty. Although these are unfortunate aspects regularly connected with the practice, I want to make it clear how barefootism from a fruitarian perspective differs. It may be true that the barefootism associated with the city homeless, often those with mental health issues, or drug or alcohol problems, or just outright poverty (caused by the underlying mentioned issues), is a reluctant situation, where practitioners have regularly also lost some or all sense of personal hygiene. Fruitarian barefootism, on the other hand, is a joyous lifestyle option, based on complete freedom of choice, spiritual grounding and a strong desire for mental and physical personal cleansing.

Years ago, back when I myself was a shackled and shod omnivore, by the end of a normal day's play or work, I would remove my shoes unleashing a terribly unpleasant foot odour in the process. There were times when I would carry one or even two extra pairs of socks with me, and change them throughout the day. My feet would get sweaty as well as stinky, and they often felt quite uncomfortable after a day of shoes. This is by no means an uncommon problem, shoes of any shape or form will all gradually and inevitably lead to foot health consequences of some form or another.

"And forget not that the Earth delights to feel your bare feet and the winds long to play with your hair."- Kahlil Gibran

True, walking bare foot may mean the occasional glass shard or thorn splinter, and if done with the wrong frame of mind, may sometimes result in the odd cut or so, especially so for newbies, but over time, as the soles of our feet regain their natural supple firmness, such occurrences will always lessen. Besides, not using footwear will also encourage us to have a greater awareness of what's in front of us, and how and where we

133

place our feet, thus rendering it far less likely to step onto, or into, something unpleasant or living. Barefootism quietens one's inner thoughts, clears one's mind and helps one to focus on the here and now, allowing one to pay attention to every step one takes.

I have been cautioned on numerous occasions, about walking barefoot through the bush; aren't I afraid of snakes? Shouldn't I wear shoes just in case? Such admonishments although naturally well meaning also show a clear lack of understanding of barefoot benefits. There was this one time, at band camp, that I did so happen to stand on the tail of a snake hidden in the grass. Because I was barefoot, I immediately felt that my foot was pushing onto something living, and thus immediately recoiled to see the snake slither away from me. Had I been wearing the heavy walking boots people get so obsessed with, it is quite likely that I would have stepped with full force onto the animal's tail, which could then likely have hurt and enraged him enough, for him to part with some of his venom. As it happens, the majority of snake bites are between the ankle and knee, so unless one wears knee or thigh length boots, it's unlikely that in such situations snakebite would be avoided.

> Walking barefoot strengthens and stretches the muscles, tendons and ligaments in your feet, ankles and calves. This helps prevent injury, knee strain and back problems. Not only that, but because it works muscles not used when you're wearing shoes, it strengthens and stretches your core, helping maintain both your balance and posture.

Letter to Librarian

Back in 2002-ish, I found myself in Glastonbury, England. I'd heard the local library was a good place to get free internet, so would occasionally visit for an hour or two. One day, while visiting, one of the librarians approached me, and asked me politely to please not come in barefoot any more. She said it was dangerous, there could be glass, that feet were dirty and that small children sometimes crawled on the carpet.

I felt this was an odd request, considering I was quite sure I had seen other barefooters in there previously (Glastonbury probably has the highest percentage of barefooters in England), but decided not to object there and then.

Instead, I left the library and wrote her a letter:

Dear Library Lady,

Hallo. I don't want you to feel bad about asking I wear shoes.

I accept that your request, although, I believe personally, based on false knowledge, was really, well-meaning.

> "You know you're old when someone compliments you on your alligator shoes and you're barefoot" - Phyllis Diller

Truthfully, I have not worn footwear since the early half of the 1990s. I have travelled across much of the European continent; by bike and on foot, as well as various other parts of the world. Rarely have I, in the course of that time, experienced anything more than the very infrequent splinter.

I don't own my own footwear and have borrowed the sandals I'm wearing, in order to walk across eight metres of carpet that we both know is well cleaned and without shards of glass. Besides I can assure you that being barefoot, one has far greater awareness of where one places one's feet.

With the cleanliness issue: In comparison to the soles of most people's footwear, my feet are far cleaner. Feelings of dirty, sweaty feet are based on feet cooped up inside socks and footwear all day, which, in such clammy, awkward, restricting environments, will naturally be a thriving breeding ground for bacteria and manufacturing of undesirably unpleasant odours.

Walking barefoot is part of my pilgrimage which has temporarily brought me to Glastonbury. It is about grounding oneself and regaining contact with mother earth. It is about permanent reflexology. The health of feet will gradually deteriorate over a lifetime of footwear (ab)usage. Tinea between the toes and other bacterial fungal infections will almost inevitably develop and most people will have deformed feet and other foot problems in their later years caused by shoes.

> In dietary terms, being shod is rather similar to cooking one's feet, as opposed to barefoot being raw.

I am not drunk, loud nor otherwise obnoxious. If I choose to let my hair grow unhindered and my beard go wild, this is basically Essenic in nature and I trust my appearance has not caused prejudgement of my character as is sometimes the case.

For these reasons and also because I have recently spoken with several other people who regularly visit the library sans foot attire, none of whom ever having been asked to don shoes, I would kindly ask that you reconsider allowing me to do so.

Kind regards, in love and light,

Mango

The next day, I borrowed a pair of sandals, I went to the library, put them on in the entry hallway and went over and sat in my favourite corner. I read some, then as I left, I handed her the letter.

I didn't see her for a week or two, but I went in there one day and she came across to me and said she'd like a word.

She told me that she'd shown the manager my note and they'd both agreed that I could come in barefoot. I was so pleased. Even sitting down with sandals on, for that short time, my feet were feeling increasingly uncomfortable.

> "Your feet walk upon the Earth and through this your spirit is connected to the universe. Our feet are our contact with the Earth and the energies that flow through it." - Cherokee "Moonmaiden" Jenny Wallace

Permanent Reflexology

Back when my feet would be regularly cooped up throughout the day, I can attest that, if the shoes were comfortable and cushioned enough, walking would seem to be so too, however, at the end of every day, my feet would inevitably feel wasted and worn. The reverse is true for me now. I feel every step I make, whether it be across hot tarmac, or rough bush terrain, I am aware of every step. Gravel, stony ground, twigs and unevenness, hot sands, sometimes to be sure a step might hurt slightly, certainly far more than any

> "Walk as if you are kissing the Earth with your feet." - Thich Nhat Hanh

usual step in shoes would, but at the end of the day, my feet generally feel great, they're odourless and considerably cleaner than they ever were when shod. It's as if I've tapped into free permanent reflexology/foot-zone therapy!

*"When you walk with naked feet,
how can you ever forget the earth?"*
- Carl Jung

NATURISM

Nudism

Mention Naturism and likely the first thing that springs to the minds of many is bare bottoms running around. There is no denying that nudism is indeed an intricate part of what naturism is about, however the two terms are by no means identical in meaning. Unlike nudism, which is basically the practice of going around naked as much as possible, naturism implies also a deep desire to seek out and enjoy more natural settings. To swim in clean, fresh flowing water, rivers, streams, lakes and ocean. To be massaged by waterfalls, to lie naked in the sun and feel its gentle caress. It implies a desire to escape civilisation, all the fumes, pollution and concrete and to enjoy and live a more back to basics lifestyle.

Nudism does not imply being constantly naked, but is instead about dropping preconceived society influenced notions of nudity being in some way shameful. It's about letting go of the fear and thtopping being tho clothed-minded. If you break a bone and have it plastered to prevent further injury, you'll know the skin under that cast, through being starved of the freedom of fresh air and sunlight, will slowly atrophy. The nerve synapses will diminish to a whimper of their former glory and the muscles will gradually weaken due to strangled restricted motion. As modern day Homosapiens there is an overwhelming tendency to shroud our entire skin palette, except for face, neck and hands, effectively obliterating health nourishing symbiosis with the planet. We hide in cocoons, when we could be free as butterflies!

"Fake people have an image to maintain. Real people just don't care." - Hikigaya Hachiman

A 2003 University of Reading study entitled "A Naked Ape Would Have Fewer Parasites"[100] posits that "humans evolved hairlessness to reduce parasite loads, especially ectoparasites that may carry disease." Unfortunately, the restrictive clothes we don can be a breeding ground for foul fungi and bad bacterium, causing yeast infections, urinary tract infections and more. Cinched-up belts, ties and elasticated clothing impede breathing. Men's snugly fitted underpants raise testicle temperature, lowering sperm count and fertility. I'm sure the list continues.

Furthermore, health benefits of social nudity include stress reduction, satiation of curiosity about the human body, reduction of porn addiction, a sense of full-body integration and developing a wholesome attitude about the opposite gender. Research at the University of Northern Iowa discovered nudists have significantly higher body self-acceptance[101],while a somewhat similar study[102] concluded teens at a New York nudist camp were "extraordinarily well-adjusted, happy and thoughtful." It's also excellent for children to grow up free of shame about the human body. Yet another study of 384 participants[103] concluded pro-nudity students "were significantly more accepting of other religious groups and gays and lesbians" when compared to the anti-nudity students. They were also "less prejudiced towards ethnically dissimilar others."

Yes, we surely live in a prudishly warped world, full of petty hangups and issues, where nudism is generally shied away from, ridiculed and frequently considered a perversion practised solely by sexual deviants.

> Don't try and justify your mistakes. When you make one, admit it, laugh at it, learn from it and above all make whatever changes are needed to correct it!

The True Perverts

An Eden Fruitarian is able to see past such uncivilised beliefs and recognises the true perversion inherent within such thinking. He understands nudity as an open integral component of Eden, ultimately unashamedly innocent, and embraces the concept with the shamelessness of a child.

Clothing is a strange concept. Especially this warped sense of "Smart" that accompanies it, based on what some rich Italian fashion designer may think best. Men who unquestioningly and habitually tie ropes around their necks (ties) and women in starchy dresses with fleckless, overly pronounced creases. Facial growth never allowed to develop. I always thought and still do, of this whole idea of "smart" as nothing short of bizarre at best.

Admittedly, though it seems now to be a life time ago, I did try to fit in for a while. I played around with the idea, three-piece pinstripe suits, the daily telegraph tucked neatly under one armpit, with an ever visible, half filled crossword and similar. I think I managed that for about a year or so, before growing tired of the charade. Although I did try, I was never really one able to fully embrace the notion and always felt like I was an imposter, looking odd at the best of times. Rather like a punked up rooster with socks. Even as a kid I used to resent it when my parents would say on a Sunday, "put your smart clothes on". I would always do so reluctantly muttering "But I'll get them dirty and you'll get upset with me!". The inevitable reply was "no we won't, don't be silly!" and the inevitable outcome, was that we'd go to the park, I'd end up with grass on my knees, and: "Oh just look at your knees!". What use is life if you aren't allowed to get your knees dirty in the grass?

People can freely choose to look this so-called "smart" if they desire. The concept of smartliness holds no appeal for me. Nowadays I'm in to minimal clothing. The ultimate ideal would be to rid myself of clothes altogether; to abandon them with complete non-attachment. Climate and society dictate otherwise though, so I practise only whenever victimisation is off the table.

> "Be a light unto the world, and hurt it not. Seek to build not destroy. Bring My people home"- Neale Donald Walsch

I recall while travelling through Malaysia in the early 2000s, sitting on a bus in the middle of nowhere in particular. It was hot out there, but judging by the apparel of the locals, one may have easily been deceived otherwise! Covered up neatly, thick denim jeans and baseball caps. Long sleeved shirts sticking sweatily to their backs. How long has it been this way? Why are we all such prudes? I don't care how my body looks, I'll gladly bare it anywhere if it means eating some sun and doesn't result in ridicule, harassment or punishment.

Rather similar to the footwear issue mentioned in the previous chapter, many so called "smart" people mistakenly equate "non smartness" with uncleanliness/dirtiness. This need not be the case at all, as the Eden Fruitarian is in many ways quite concerned with hygiene and cleanliness. Just not via means of soaps, shampoos or toothpastes. I believe profoundly that cleanliness is next to Godliness and that smartliness and cleanliness have nothing to do with each other. If only smart people were really smart and could see their insides! They are generally like heavily decorated houses that look overly sparkling and glamorous on the outsides, while their insides are rodent infested mounds of discarded dirty old socks, covered in kitchen grease, dustballs and piles of forsaken washing up. Ha! Hippy bathday to you!

Soaps and Shampoos

Yes, in desiring to get back to nature, it should become clear to those who give it thought enough, that items such as soaps, detergents, cleansing powders, make-up and more, hold no real value. It's funny how we associate soap with cleanliness, seeing as soap in and of itself is so "not" clean. It is pretty much always highly processed and generally full of non-existent naturally occurring chemicals, concentrated in profusion. Most soaps include also some ingredients from the animal industry too. E.g., gelatine. Water sullied with soaps and so called cleaning products, dirty and pollute the earth. Natural earth on the other hand is fun and, contrary to what we've been brainwashed into thinking, cleansing. A good mud bath can cool you down in the heat of the day and really cleanse those pores better than most every soap.

Time flies like an arrow.
Fruit flies like a pineapple.

I stopped using soap in the mid 1980s and began instead to rely purely water. Shortly after that, I quit using shampoo too and ceased also using detergents and other household cleaning products, including washing powders. Ceasing the use of shampoos was the most difficult. I guess the hair becomes addicted, it seems to begin craving it. But after just a few weeks, the head somehow adjusts to the lack of the presence of shampoo and things normalise again. I really believe soap is detrimental to the skin, ageing it prematurely by robbing it of natural oils and subjecting it to whatever chemicals are contained within the soap.

Nudists are people who
wear suits with one button!

I know many readers might argue its case, stating there are environmentally friendly soaps, or sometimes you might believe the only way to get rid of something is with a soap or a heavy detergent of some kind. But the reality is probably that so called environmentally friendly soaps are just not as polluting as the other more commercially available one's. Sure, the original raw ingredients may theoretically be relatively harmless, but is the harvesting of them? Or the process they undergo? And what effect will polluted water have when returned to the soil or into water ways?

As for those times when you're having difficulties with stains, I say, think twice before bleaching. Leave the stain be. Don't let yourself be ruled by fashion or by false senses of smartliness. Every stain gives the clothing history!

Toothpastes are often employed to disguise the bad breaths originating from bad diets. Eat properly and any need to cover up one's internal body odours with minty fresh pastes will vanish.

Sun Creams

Sunshine is not your enemy!

We have been told how sun creams prevent skin cancer. Indeed, society encourages its use whenever we spend extended periods of time in the sun. Some refusing to leave the house without it.

My personal view point is one of extreme scepticism toward this supposed beneficial usage of sunscreen. Actually, perversely enough, I really believe the reverse may be true, and that sun creams may themselves be partially responsible for evoking sun cancer. Put aside what you have been told, what is generally accepted as being fact and ponder over the following: Sun creams contain a whole host of chemicals which are far from natural. In fact, some of the ingredients in sun creams have been demonstrated to be carcinogenic (actually promoting the *devil-upment* of cancer cells!).

Actually, just reading the labels makes me feel queasy. Isotridecyl salicylate, Octyl salicylate, Butyl methoxydibenzoylmethane. Need I go on?

Sun on the other hand, is totally natural, and without it all creatures on this planet, likely even all life, would end. It gives us a steady supply of Vitamin D (whatever that is!), which is believed by many to be crucial for the absorption of Calcium in the body, but from a naturist, barefoot fruitarian's perspective, the most important thing we need to understand is how, providing we don't over do it, the sun just feels plain great!

"Never tell a young person that anything cannot be done. God may have been waiting centuries for someone ignorant enough of the impossible to do that very thing." - John A. Holmes

Skin, along with one's kidneys, intestines, liver and lungs (S.K.I.L.L), is a major organ of elimination, meaning some of what we detox, emerges through the skin. It is my belief that the sun's caress is of vital importance to help cleanse the skin of surface toxins. By applying oil and chemical based sun creams to our skin, we are affectively hindering the skin from detoxing and in addition, actually absorbing new chemicals through the skin pores from the lotions themselves.

141

At some stage on the Eden Fruitarian path, you will begin to know through increased olfactory awareness, just how toxic sun creams really are. The toxic stenches of the beach going masses who spread it sickly thickly onto their poor toxin overloaded bodies is at times quite overpowering.

During the heat of the summer, after gradually letting more and more sunshine onto my body, I find I can be outside most of the day and rarely do I get burnt. Sometimes I find my nose is a bit of a weak point, and will keep it covered to prevent too much skin flaking off. Should it happen that we get burnt, we just apply a little aloe vera, fresh from its leaf.

We also enjoy massaging fruit peel into the skin (especially papaya or mango!) and find that really helps the skin to not get burned too.

Not convinced? Read further: [104]

Hair

"Give me a head with hair, long beautiful hair. Shining, gleaming steaming, flaxen, waxen. Give me it down to there. Hair, shoulder length or longer, here baby, there mamma, everywhere daddy, daddy hair! Flow it, show it, long as God can grow it, my hair" ♫- From Musical Hair

In seeing the folly of the concrete jungle, with its accompanying peer pressured insanities, it should make us stop up and question pretty much everything. Society tries to hammer the wildness out of us and turn us all into sheeple like drones who follow unquestioningly. One expression of that conformity is through taming our hair, we might think we are expressing our individuality through shaving it all off, ironing it flat, perming it all frizzy like, or dying it pink with blue stripes, but these are all encouraged practices that generally ultimately serve to grease the wheels of the concrete economy.

I didn't like my beard at first, then it grew on me.

The Eden Fruitarian dispenses with such ingrained conditioning and the thought that hair styling is in some way important, and finally lets his hairs grow naturally, however they so choose. Along with chaetophobia[105], pogonophobia[106] is completely absent, and if one's beard decides to reach for the belly button, then so be it! Make it so!

I was reading an article[107] online recently that indicated how long unhindered hair may in some way be connected to a sixth sense. The article described how during the Vietnam War, experts were sent out to find Native Americans who were blessed with uncanny, seemingly

142

supernatural, abilities to track.

A couple of American Indians were selected. What followed will be surprising to many. Once they were recruited, their natural skills and ability to access their sixth sense just disappeared. On conducting a test to find out what went wrong, the older native American recruits said that after undergoing military haircut, they could no longer sense the enemy, they lost their intuition power and were no longer able to access subtle extrasensory information.

> "I don't advice a haircut man, all hairdressers are in the employment of the government, hair are your aerials, they pick up signals from the cosmos and transmit them directly into the brain. This is the reason bald headed men are so uptight"
> - Danny from "Withnail and I"

So more native Indians were recruited and this time they were allowed to keep their hair long. On comparing performance of men with a standard military haircut and ones with long hair, they discovered that long-haired men were far more skilful. The results stated that the Native trackers should be allowed to keep their hair long.

I can't help but wonder how they may also have been affected through relinquishing contact with the earth, and being forced to wear boots!

Long hair has long been a common element of many spiritual prophets such as Jesus, Moses, Buddha and Shiva. Likely many of us can recall too, the story of Samson and Delilah from the Bible, when Samson lost his strength with the loss of his hair.

It appears that hair may in some way be an extension of the nervous system. If this is true, then when hair is cut, receiving and sending transmissions to and from the environment will surely be hampered.

Temple Graffiti

> My body is a temple, therefore I now declare myself TAX EXEMPT!

Our bodies should be seen as temporary sacred temples of the soul and our duty to keep our individual one clean. Both internally and externally. Internally this is done by eating the right food; fruit. Thus avoiding any foods that sludge and sully the interior (especially animal products and cooked foods of any kind!). Externally, regular bathes in water will normally suffice, but all fruits can also be massaged into the skin with benefits. The skins of mangos and papaya feel especially pleasant, as does a head/hair bath in lemon juice[108]. Let them soak in for at least ten minutes before gently washing off with natural water (preferably non chlorinated, and non fluoridated), you will feel the benefit!

The Eden Fruitarian sees the sacrilegious idiocy of defacing one's external temple walls through carving tattoo patterns and shapes onto them. He has no desire to vandalise the temple through puncturing holes around, through and into it, nor to adorn it with metal rings, chains and studs. Even the less harsh graffiti of make-up is recognised as being detrimental to the skin and thus to be avoided at all cost, and the idea of artificially odourising oneself through the use of perfumes and the like, as quite repulsive. The Huffington Post has an article about a woman who wears make-up for a month without washing it off[109]. The skin ageing affect is quite alarming, see for yourself, but the only conclusion really pushed is to make sure you wash it off each evening. Such short-sightedness! No amount of creams and pastes and make-up will make you look better than you do already! Stop with the lack of self confidence, recognise your own beauty. Unleash it! The paints do nothing but accentuate your lack of inner strength.

The mere notion that the body should be tampered with through the completely inessential utilisation of cosmetic surgery is even more sickening. We are all born beautiful and if we have lost that beauty through the constant sullying and scumming of our internal organs, the only real way to regain it, is to set upon the, perhaps long and often arduous journey, of cleansing it and restoring it to the health of our given birthright, which we have chosen unwittingly to trash.

> "Naked came I out of my mother's womb and naked shall I return there: the Lord gave and the Lord has taken away; may the name of the Lord be blessed." - Job 1:21

Of course, awakening to Eden Fruitarianism can occur at any stage of one's life and we will all have a history before arriving there. If it should so happen that yours included the piercings, the tattoos and the regular daily appliance of skin and hair paints to enhance or cover up certain features you have deemed not good enough and been unhappy with, then just accept this was history. There is no point in giving yourself a hard time about things you were ignorant of, just learn from your mistakes. If the damage you have done is irreversible, just accept that you've erred and commit yourself to not doing so again, or at least to attempt to not do so again.

PET PEEVES

I've written of how we need to change our attitudes toward species other than our own. How we need to stop seeing them as food, and start respecting them as individuals. Indeed I am guessing it is likely clear to most readers that animals have no desire to be imprisoned and murdered for their flesh and skins. It should be clear too, no animal will be happy to be confined and experimented upon, as is the plight of those suffering vivisection. Equally, the whole concept of animal circuses and "zooillogical" gardens should be recognised as fundamentally exploitive of all animals involved.

> "The whole future of the Earth depends on the awakening of our faith in the future."
> - Pierre Teilhard de Chardin

As a quick side note, I just want to congratulate certain countries on recognising the inappropriateness of animal abuse in entertainment. There is a slowly awakening global realisation, and several countries are forbidding the use of animals in both circuses[110] and even zoos[111]!

What many will also tend, or choose, to be unaware of though, is the exploitation of the animals right under their very noses. I am talking of course of the Rexes, Tabbies, Scruffies, Sooties, Snowies, Sheps, Gingers, Misties, Oscars and Rovers among us.

From an Eden Fruitarian perspective, there is little to zero justification for continuing the practice of keeping companion animals, or pets as they are more colloquially referred to as. The way I see it, the vast majority of pets are only companions for as far as it suits their owner's needs and comfort. Even the whole concept of "owning" someone else I find rather sickening and to be sure, it *is* a legal "ownership" we are talking of here. There is a clear master and a clear servant, even if some pet owners frequently joke that these roles are reversed.

Cats and dogs, probably making up the bulk of the companion animal market, are forcibly removed from their broods, litters and families, exchanging hands rather like slaves once did between humans, often by a business or individual who reaps financial reward through the transaction and **never** with full concern for the animals own true needs, comforts and desires. I have no doubt that in many cases, both offspring and parents are left traumatised through the experience, if only for brief periods of time during transition. Of course, humans will make all manner of excuses and justifications, that they fully believe they are somehow doing the animal a favour and offering her a good, warm, loving home, where the animal will be fed, pampered, appreciated and otherwise well taken care of.

The truth though, is the keeping of animals is pretty much always exploitative of the animals in question. They are there because their keepers have chosen to have them there, and rarely because they themselves have consciously chosen their environment. Thus, the predominant reason for keeping pets is clearly a selfish one. Throughout their imprisoned lives, the vast majority of companion animals are left to spend hours alone. Dogs often driven to temporary or even permanent insanity through boredom and loneliness, barking incessantly for hours on end, at any untoward noises. The owners are often fully oblivious to the dog's failing mental welfare, as our canine friends have an innate capability for forgiveness and will generally immediately become overly happy and enthused on the return of an absent master who has been gone all day.

Honestly, can we truthfully say we deserve such loyalty, faithfulness and forgiveness? Isn't this really just an example of how we exploit these animals for our own selfish ends? With human companions we have to work out our relationships, knowing we may not be forgiven for whatever we do and that we cannot simply take without giving anything in return.

> Tradition should never be reasoning enough to continue any practice. Acts must be seen for what they are and not for what we are told they might be. Cannibalism has been accepted tradition in many places (why restrict ourselves to our own traditions!) - Tradition is a poor excuse at the best of times.

Cats generally have a fairer deal as in many ways they are more independent than dogs and can be trusted to be alone outside for the bulk of the day, but they too are very much enslaved and ultimately degraded through their dependency on humans. It is humans who decide what, when and where they can eat and, exercising our dominance over them, we frequently have them physically mutilated such that they are no longer able to procreate. Dogs we have even more control over, deciding when and where they get their free time, exercise and play and who and which other species they are allowed to interact with. We drag them around on leashes, only let them poo and pee when we feel the time and place are fitting and angrily bark and snarl instructions at them when they do what comes natural to them and disobey or behave in ways fitting of a dog.

Actually, I just wrote that cats can be trusted to be alone outside all day, but well, that trust can only be extended toward their encounters with larger species as many a small urban wildlife falls victim of the currently natural hunting instincts of domestic cats. But I intend to get to more on this later in my next chapter on NATURE.

The truth is too, from a vegan perspective, cats and dogs are often fed diets consisting predominantly of the flesh of other animals. Now if you call yourself vegan and truly understand the guidelines of being a vegan, how can you possibly rationalise such actions?

How Many Animals to Feed Your Dog?

I read once, somewhere, in a vegan magazine maybe, probably back in the late 1980s, rough statistics someone had knocked together about how much an average dog of an average size might eat throughout the course of an average doggy lifetime. I wish I had cut out the article, as I believe its fundamental reasoning was pretty soundly logical and to the point. The facts were laid bare and the statistics showed that such an average canine could eat the equivalent of one cow, three sheep, three pigs, a hundred chickens and countless fish and of course a fair bit of veggies and grains too, irrelevant to the current thought experiment. The numbers given here are purely my own fantasy, as I see no real point in calculating things more precisely. Whether it's one hundred chickens, twenty or five hundred, makes little difference, the truth remains the same though, whatever the actual figures may be, if you think you are helping animals by keeping a dog and feeding him a traditional canned diet, then think again. By doing so you are contributing toward making the lives of many other individuals living hells.

> Lock your spouse and a dog in a car for five hours, and when you get back, see which one of them will be happy to see you!

Of course, dogs can be fed vegan diets and are said to fair exceptionally well on such. In fact, I also recall reading some years ago, that the worlds oldest living dog at the time was in fact vegan and eating much of her food raw too. Brambles was her name and I read later she died in 2003, pushing 28 she was[112]. (That would have made her well over 190 in dog years!)

Converting your dog to vegan will naturally help to relieve the bloodshed on the planet and our over abusive nature toward animals, but considering not trading in further potential animals after the dog passes over, will aid yet further.

Cats it seems have a more difficult time existing on a vegan diet, and I'm told success is only achievable via synthetic taurine (a protein they apparently cannot live well without). Although the statistics for what a cat might eat throughout an average life are likely somewhat less than the average dog, the figures would nevertheless still be comparable. The way I see it, keeping cats, especially and veganism and particularly Eden Fruitarianism, are just not compatible. If you don't find yourself being forced into a compromise and buying the butchered flesh of other animals, then you'll still have the issue of the spaying neutering and likely consequential loss of birds and similar small wildlife from your back yard, which are partially your responsibility. (by some estimates, over three billion birds are killed annually by cats![113])

Companion animals have dependency thrust upon them. Before Eden can become a reality, it is crucial we do whatever we can to give them back their independence.

Unfortunately, like shoes, many people have cat and dog fetishes, where they believe they are loving owners but in reality fail to see the full picture. Even to the point where they claim to love their pets more than their husbands, wives or own children. It surely seems to me like something must be wrong there.

Of course, cats and dogs are not the only animals kept as pets, some fair far worse. Fish confined to small tanks for the amusement of guests and owners alike, birds never allowed to stretch their wings imprisoned in cages, or if allowed out, often to have their wings forcibly periodically clipped. Out of curiosity, I picked up some fish food flake thing recently and looked at the ingredients and even that wasn't vegan! It had powdered fish in it!

Then of course there are the hamster, mice and other rodents people enslave for life and less common lizards, snakes and other reptiles too. None of whom ever get a truly fair deal.

If you think you are doing an animal a favour by rescuing him from a pound, then you are doing countless others an injustice. By doing so you help perpetuate the collective thought that keeping companion animals is normal and as soon as your animal is removed from the pound, it will be replaced. I'm afraid I'm with Spock on this one, and think that the needs of the many far outweigh the needs of the one, and as long as we keep on supporting this pet industry, the bloody pounds will continue to exist. It's a vicious circle, which can only be brought to an end by going off on a tangent and washing our hands of it.

A Horsey Story

Just recently I ran into an acquaintance at our local market. She and her family keep horses as pets. Her husband was throwing

> Trying to reason with some people, is like trying to play chess with a pigeon.

snide comments around about meat eaters and their ilk, and how he wouldn't trust to have them on their land for fear of their horses being eaten. Now I understood he wasn't being totally realistic with his scenario, but for some reason it really rubbed me up the wrong way and I immediately began questioning why it was they kept horses in the first place. Not liking my question, the husband left pretty much immediately, leaving myself and his wife to discuss the topic in more detail.

Now, bearing in mind they are self declared raw vegans, and quite outspoken at that, her justifications seemed pretty bizarre. To begin with, her major argument appeared to revolve around a supposed fact that to be honest I had hitherto never heard of, nor consequently given any thought to. Apparently, she began telling me, horses are unique in that they, and they alone among species, have a gap between two different sets of teeth, and that therefore horses must have been created by God to be faithful companions to humans, as the gap was a perfect fit for the bit[d]. To me this response was comparable to the meat eater who defends meat eating by saying "Animals must have been created by God for us to eat, otherwise they wouldn't taste so good". You can't really argue with that one.

> Definition of Stupid: Knowing the truth, seeing the truth, but still believing the lies.

She continued, stating a horse's back was perfectly designed for humans to sit upon and supposed that in the garden of Eden, we would ride our trusty steeds at exhilarating speeds through the orchards to get much sought after adrenalin rushes and reach fruit three kilometres away. I'm guessing her version of Eden wouldn't be exciting enough for her without them. Frankly I found her opinions at first to be rather vexing, in that they didn't really seem to make much sense to me. I countered by informing her that wild horses

---

d   A mouthpiece, typically made of metal, that is attached to a bridle and used to control a horse.

naturally don't mix with humans and will do their best to avoid them. In fact, the only way horses can be exploited as we do, is through a lengthy painful humiliating breaking in process, which she somehow managed to believe was irrelevant as that had happened generations ago.

Actually, later on when I got home, I felt a need to get online and verify her statement about horses being the only animals with that gap. I doubted its authenticity and after wielding my trusty google, soon discovered that cows and most other ruminants have the gap which is called the "interdental gap". In fact, zebras and donkeys have them too. A little further research showed me, and the percentages vary depending on which website I looked at, but somewhere between 50 to 80% of horses (as opposed to, from what I can tell, 0% of cattle!) actually do grow teeth in the interdental gap. Something called "Wolf teeth" and if they are allowed to grow, would make the usage of a "bit" extremely uncomfortable, even painful. Thus equine dentists are routinely called in to remove them.

> Everyone wants to be a rational thinker and yet no one wants to think rationally!

I am guessing that, as this lady and her family have six or seven horses, they would likely have been aware of this fact and thus in justification of their animal dominance outlook, deliberately did not disclose the full truth.

Discussing this further with Květa, she and I reflected on the supposition that a horses back was designed for humans to sit on, and Květa pointed out if that were true, people wouldn't need to create and use saddles to make the ride more comfortable. So true.

I find this kind of attitude actually quite typical of pet owners. People have attachments toward their pets, whatever animal species they may belong to, and God forbid should anyone dare challenge that attachment.

What I find odd though, is rather like with regards to diet, where people consider some species fair game and others off limit, with no particular logic behind their conclusions, people have a tendency to view other species off limit in terms of companion animal options too. Take the discussion about the horses. I made a quite logical comparison toward keeping chimpanzees as pets, as opposed to the keeping of horses. Proposing a similar scenario where a theoretical chimpanzee family had been in captivity for an already given number of generations and had thus lost all his wildness and would even seek out the company of other humans, preferring time spent with them, their company, affection and food shared with them, over even the eventual sometimes given available freedom of the outdoors. I asked if she would consider that having such an animal as a companion would be acceptable, but she refused to go there and, clearly a little offended, informed me that "horses are unique" and that such a comparison was invalid and that the gap was categorical proof. I countered that chimpanzees were unique too, indeed, all animal species are unique. Shucks, even all individual members of each species are unique.

In retrospect, I think I should have chosen zebras or cows as my comparison animals (especially had I been aware that these animals shared the supposedly unique to horses interdental gap!). And one could well imagine that these animals also, over time, could have their wills broken, wild and untamed spirits subdued and become servitude to humans. I guess I just wasn't thinking fast enough.

Anyhow, there was a lesson in their for me too, as I came away feeling agitated and unsettled and know it was because my whole attitude had been wrong, and getting wired and fired up about issues which ultimately were beyond my control was not productive for anyone.

> "Stagnation is death. If you don't change, you die. It's that simple. It's that scary." - Leonard Sweet

Seeing the Full Picture

Likely there are many who have bought animals in the past, who would find this whole chapter offensive to them, believing that I'm not seeing the full picture, when to be honest, I feel I see it far more clearly than most.

I guess many might counter that some animals have been domesticated over centuries, so this somehow justifies the perpetuation of such dominance, but personally I don't fathom how this should mean it is right to continue such perverse customs. Slavery was once widely practised in the past, but is today just as widely condemned.

As for animals choosing to live closely to us, I'm anthropomorphising again, but as a species I'm guessing they did not expect to have to give up their freedom and the world was a very different place back when it all began. Humans themselves were living in Low-Tech, close to nature ways, not in cities with motor cars and central heating and canned pet food.

I like to believe humans will evolve their consciousnesses, realising pets are not a natural addition to one's family, and that the pet industry will eventually see its demise. The only animals who have complete freedom and autonomy are wild animals.

I understand the occasional companionship of a non-human animal is said to have therapeutic value, but so can that of a human, and it is because we have isolated the aged and disabled, and no longer live in small close knit tribal communities, that the need for such company arises. Even better company would be another loving sympathetic human companion. Of course, having a human or animal friend is not exactly comparable, I see that, but I refer again to the "everlasting" ability of a dog to "forgive" (no matter what you have done!) and to remain loyal, that may be true, but do we really deserve that? What do we learn if we are continuously forgiven for mistreating and abusing others?

> You can trust your dog to guard your house, but never to guard your sandwich.

Robot Pets

As a side note, and as a possible future relief for pet people, I hear the Japanese are making progress in creating robot pets that may one day replace our fellow sentient beings as faithful domestic companions[114]. This I see as far from ideal, but at least it could mean animals cease being exploited for the purpose. This would be somewhat like synthetic meat to the newbie vegetarians, or soy cheese to the lasagne craving vegan!

Sexual Mutilation

The fact that the majority of pets are spayed or neutered should be a deal breaker for many budding opening awarenesses, the sexual mutilation is often more to do with maintaining our control over their lives, than any real concern about uncontrolled cross breeding and is another predicament that we have gotten into by keeping animals as pets. Spaying and neutering animals is committing gross acts of violence against them. A clear question of animal rights. Spaying and neutering denies animals the right to mate, to be parents, to have families of their own. If you somehow think the end justifies the means, tell me how complacent you would be, to be forcibly neutered, or how *right* you think it would be, to forcibly mass neuter humans in overpopulated areas of the earth?

Whilst the present attitude toward pets continues, Dog Homes will never run out of animals. Only a small percentage of abandoned and ill-treated animals are ever rescued and, here's an interesting statistic, over one thousand homeless dogs are slaughtered weekly by the UK RSPCA alone! Likely a fair percentage of them will themselves end up as pet food[115]. I quote: *"Many of these animals* [that end up in pet feed] *died after being medicated for health problems that contributed to their deaths, and not all drugs are neutralized during the rendering process. Meat and bone meal can contain antibiotics, steroids, and even the sodium pentobarbital used to kill pets at shelters. By definition, a lot of the animals that ended up in the rendering vat had something wrong with them.."* This is food which is considered unfit for human consumption that is often unquestioningly fed to companion animals.

There is no compassionate way forward that includes enslaving animals, unless these animals are completely autonomous, free to come and go as they choose, to be with their own kinds if they wish and to do all the things wild animals do.

The best way that children can learn to respect, love and value non-human animals is to see them and learn about them in their free

> Remember lights shine their brightest when turned on in the darkness.

and natural state. Having pets does not teach respect for animals. If that were true, all pet owners would be vegan!

I understand every situation is different, and there are cases where animals may choose us too. I've been fortunate enough to experience this on more than one occasion, and can vouch that there is a great joy to be had in gaining the trust of a wild animal. In such situations, I believe we should feel privileged and blessed when wild animals choose to befriend us, and not desire to take advantage of their trust.

The term "pet" is disputed by some, concerning their own choice(s) of companion animals. My colleagues with the horses would likely never call them pets, but, well, it's just semantics and by definition a pet is a domesticated animal kept for companionship and/or amusement and I certainly see this as the predominant reason they are keeping horses. If the horses never sought out their company, refused to let them approach or mount and ride them, shied away from them, keeping to themselves at the back of their land, I seriously doubt they would ever consider reinvesting in new ones. Actually I've since witnessed how their horses are kept mostly penned in or tied to stakes for long periods, and realise just how much denial there was in the "horses running freely scenario" she had described to me.

Animal Lovers

It's an unfortunate reality that many pet owners mistakenly consider themselves to be animal lovers, indeed, I recall a survey where participants were questioned whether or not they believed in animal rights. Quite a high percentage answered yes. It turned out though, they had believed the question related purely to dogs and cats. For them, being an animal lover means loving their shitzu poodle and thinking nothing of eating a heart(attack)y egg and bacon breakfast.

> You can't truthfully claim to love animals and yet still choose to eat them.

I occasionally feel the urge to comment on those facebook images of a dog or cat being mistreated, with the accompanying text that animal abusers need to be severely punished. You'd be surprised how emotional some commenters can get, crying out for the death penalty for those who hurt animals[116]. Not too surprisingly, whenever it is pointed out that the logical conclusion of this is to become vegan, cognitive dissonance steps in, and the most irrational answers are given that frequently make little to no sense.

Then there is the issue of toxigens in animal fur. Toxoplasma gondii is one particular parasite found on house cats which is easily transmitted to humans and can cause serious harm to the unborn foetus. Apparently it takes up residence inside the human brain and some statistics estimate as many as 50% of us are infected with it! Okay, it's said to be relatively benign, but studies have suggested there's a correlation between this parasite and several different personality traits[117].

When broaching the subject of keeping pets on my blog in the past, it was suggested by more than one reader, that I was perhaps being a little too blanket about the overall situation of pet keeping. That things aren't always as black and white as I make them out to be; that there can be mutual benefit for both the companion animal and the owner/keeper and that other animals need not consequently be slaughtered nor harmed in the process.

Okay, so let's examine such a hypothetical situation. Firstly, it is pretty clear to me that those who defend pet keeping in such a manner, are likely doing so because they themselves are attached in some fashion, to the idea of animal keeping. Secondly, although I don't altogether gainsay the possibility of such a scenario, I just see it as being highly improbable. There are always issues and situations that arise making it profoundly clear that we are still most assuredly talking of a master/servant relationship. I think, for example, we can safely rule out city kept dogs as ever fitting into such a postulated synopsis. They rarely get the free range they require and desire, and there is often the additional problem of their discordant barking disturbing what little peace there is to be had in urban settings. I'm sure most city dwellers and many country dwellers have had their sleeps disrupted with the incessant yelping of bored night-time canines. Such a contrast to the gentle chorus of frogs and crickets.

Even out in the country, where a dog gets to live with several of their own kind, and is given more or less free and unfettered range, and theoretically still, fed a vegan diet, there are a multitude of other factors to consider. Least of which is the high likelihood that the ingrained pack hunting mentality and instinct will resurface causing terror for not only local wildlife, but also for those of us who enjoy a pleasant country stroll. I've lost count of the amount of times free roaming dogs have caused me momentary fear and compelled me to change my trajectory.

And if they are not sexually mutilated and allowed to freely mingle with their own unmutilated kind, there is the concern of inevitable offspring, perpetuating the problem ad infinitum. Most people are unaware that roughly only one in ten to twelve dogs and cats ever find a home[118]. Many of the rest end up being sent to rendering stations where their carcasses are processed into, among other things, pet food. In the US alone nearly 10,000 pound animals are slaughtered daily[119]!

In a Nutshell

I'm recalling witnessing a vendor sitting outside of a Buddhist monastery in Thailand. Beside him he had a cage full of some kind of small squirrel like rodents. A likely devout Buddhist exited the temple grounds and approached this man, they exchanged a few words and the Buddhist handed him some money. The vendor reached into the cage and took out one of the small animals and let her loose on the ground. The Buddhist bowed and walked away. He'd done his good

> If you truly love animals, forget the dogs and cats; focus on the pigs and chickens!

deed for the day and freed an innocent animal, thus in the process (and I'm sure this was his logic) lessened his karmic burden. I stood by to see what would happen next. The animal, bewildered by its newly presented freedom, sat there confused looking, not knowing where to turn. The vendor, calmly grabbed her and after returning her to the cage, sat and waited for the next customer.

Now, although I'm hoping it may be clear to most reading this, that the Buddhist really did nothing to aid the plight of the imprisoned animal, in fact, if anything, he was the partial cause of the animal being imprisoned to begin with. Without him and others similarly short-sighted, the vendor would gain no financial benefit from capturing those animals and sitting there outside the monastery.

> "You cannot hang out with negative people and expect to live a positive life." - Joel Osteen

This is how I see the pet industry is kept afloat, by people who although they basically mean well, are just too short sighted to see the bigger picture. They may kid themselves that they are animal lovers and are saving the life of one animal, but the reality goes much much deeper. They are financing a trade which is riddled with animal abuse.

As for the argument from the owner who claims to love their pet more than anyone or anything else. If anything this should make one question society as it is, and one's warped idea of love. I read a story recently about a Dutch woman who regularly visited a zoo in Rotterdam[120], She went specifically to observe a particular gorilla named Bokito, believing she and the gorilla had a special connection. One day, the gorilla escaped his enclosure and with great deliberation, headed straight for the woman, who he grabbed, mauled and dragged around like a rag doll. Apparently her constant staring at him, was winding the fellow up to the point where he could no longer stand it and despite the water separating them and the fact that gorillas don't swim, in a fit of rage he just went for her.

> "A book can teach you, a conversation can assure you, a poem can seduce you, a genius can inspire you, but only you can save yourself." - Anthony Anaxagorou

I honestly think these so called animal lovers often don't really have a clue. I know the gorilla story isn't really related to the pet issue, although the concept of keeping any animal in captivity is pretty repulsive, I stand by what I say and believe that as long as this pet mentality remains, the accompanying pounds (animal concentration camps) will forever be kept open.

I am not trying to point the finger at anyone particularly, and for those who have already entered into the commitment of owning and caring for a companion animal, I don't wish for it to sound like my recommendation be for you to ditch the animal, even though, yes, I strongly believe it most likely *was* a mistake in getting him in the first place. But if that damage is done, it is our moral obligation to come to terms with it as best we are able. I only hope that some deeper thought on the subject might lead one to think twice before allowing oneself to make similar such future choices.

> If you are not convinced about this chapter, you should consult Dogless Graham. Let him tell you. He's a Doctor, so he must be right.

Respecting the Wild

Should we be privileged enough to be in regular contact with genuinely wild species of animal, it is important for any friendship with them to not revolve around them loosing their independence.

As an example, the previous tenant on the land we are now joyfully living on, began the habit of feeding the local kookaburras with butchered diced flesh. To be sure, the birds soon learned of the regular free meal thrown onto the rooftop of a utility shed and began just hanging around in anticipation.

There is no doubt the fellow meant well, but he did not realise that through befriending the kookaburras in this way, he was effectively disabling them, making them dependent and lazy. They no longer spent time looking for their own food, but would just wait around to be fed. When we moved in, they continued expecting the free meals and would call out angrily for us to feed them. For a while, the old tenant continued to come once or twice a week and throw the chopped meat onto the roof. It took us a while to realise what he was doing and putting two and two together, asked him politely to please stop.

The kookaburras went through a period of transition, where for a while they would hang around expecting once more to be fed, calling out whenever we ventured in the direction of the shed. It appeared too as if their feathers looked slightly unkempt as if they were not cleaning themselves properly.

After a while, they began to get used to searching for their own food

157

again. They still live here and wake us up each morning with their melodious laughter, but have now regained their stolen independence and once more find their own meals. (Their feathers definitely appear to be glossier now too!)

This is probably fortunate for us as there are the occasional venomous snake around, and the local kookaburra population help keep them at bay.

In 2010, we were living in a house in town, we would often be out in the small garden we had, where we grew among other things, tomatoes, cucumbers, papayas and passion fruit. A small bird would often be hanging around, a native willy wagtail, a regular guest star in suburban gardens here. I used to talk to him as I gardened and one day, he bravely flew onto my head, touched it briefly and flew off again. Over the following week or so, he did this more and more frequently, just flew up and touched me, on my arm or leg or head. It did not take long before he one day settled firmly onto my arm. I looked at him, smiled and talked to him. He flew off, but from then on, would regularly fly and land on me as I gardened.

Some days later, he also began showing such familiarity with Květa and much to her joy too, began landing on her while in the garden. He would even sit on the windowsill of the house and call out for us to come outside. After he had built his home and was the proud father of three small offspring, he called me to see the nest in the back garden mango tree. Beautifully made precision work. and three very cute babies.

We never fed the bird, so I'm supposing the relationship was purely one of friendship. This went on for about a year, we took quite a few photos of him with us. Eventually, we are guessing, the neighbour's cat might have gotten him as he completely disappeared from the garden.

> Marge: Watch out for the apple pie.
> Grandpa: Uh-ohh…
> Marge: Grandpa, did you sit on the apple pie?
> Grandpa: I sure hope so.

Pet Poop

Then there is the issue with toxicity of pet poop. Unlike many other species faeces, cats' and dogs' are particularly toxic. You never hear of people putting dog shit on their roses. The shit of flesh eaters is always more toxic than that of herbivorous animals, which is why it is not recommended for the conventional dieter to recycle their own waste in their gardens. The story is quite different for fruitarians.

Summary

OK. To summarise why we should reconsider support of the pet trade:

1. It keeps those animal species involved enslaved.
2. It necessitates the murder of many other animals.
3. It causes the murder of many other dogs and cats.
4. It causes and supports bloody sex mutilation.
5. It causes animals to be driven insane from boredom and loneliness and separation
6. It causes noise pollution, (bored dog barking).
7. It makes us think we are animal lovers when we are not. (Animal lovers don't eat animals!)
8. It restricts our own personal freedom as such animals are always dependent on us.

"Unless someone like you cares a whole awful lot,
nothing is going to get better. It's not."
- Dr. Seuss

All Companion and domesticated
animals have dampened spirits.
Compare a wild brumby[121]
(feral horses of Australia)
to a domesticated horse.
While the wild brumbies roam powerfully free,
with terrains spanning up to hundreds
of kilometres, their subdued shod counterparts
stand listlessly forgotten in fenced paddocks.
Their sparks are gone. Their spirits' blackened.
Vitalities just deranged fractions
of their potential glories.
Compare the house dog, to the wolf.
Can you not see the injustice?
Their liberties must be reinstated!

RELIGION AND SPIRITUALITY

You may have jumped to the conclusion that Eden Fruitarianism is in some way connected to a religion, especially considering Eden is such a historically biblical concept. This is far from the truth though. Eden Fruitarianism does not identify with any specific religion, cult or sect, orthodox or otherwise. Indeed, whether or not the biblical Eden ever truly existed is really irrelevant to the issue.

You may also have initially picked up this book thinking it was about diet, but that too is a false assumption. The crux of Eden Fruitarianism is really about recognising sentience, empathising with it and doing the right thing by all parties concerned.

Pushing aside very personal beliefs in Deities and fairy god mothers, if I am not mistaken, this also just so happens to be the neglected crux of all religious teachings.

The Golden Rule

"You don't need religion to have morals. If you can't determine right from wrong then you lack empathy, NOT religion." - Unknown

Yes! The profound essence of all religions is really about doing no harm, treating others with the respect we ourselves expect, or fundamentally deserve, and generally loving and helping others when and where we are able. This is what scholars have for centuries called "the Golden Rule"[122].

Buddhism, for example, has what it calls the five precepts, the first of which clearly states that **one should undertake the precept to refrain from harming all living creatures**, both humans and other life forms alike. And by inference it seems that the ultimate harm is the taking of life! I'm sure there are Buddhists who understand and act fittingly upon this tenet, but to be honest, I've yet to meet any who go out of their way to put this into practice, and I've even read that even the Dalai Lama regularly eats the flesh from other beings.

Christianity, in addition to Jesus's teachings of respect for others, has the very clear sixth commandment given in the old testament "**thou shall not kill**"

"To say that you kill in the name of God is blasphemy" - Pope Francis

(Exodus 20:13; Deuteronomy 5:17). Matthew 7:12 says it pretty clearly too with "**So in everything, do to others what you would have them do to you, for this sums up the Law and the Prophets**".

Speciesists scholars addicted to the scorched flesh of butchered animals, have tried to distort the true meaning of the sixth commandment and would have us believe that it refers purely to the murder of another human being, where as I would seriously doubt that any such exception was ever implied or intended. Some have been even more liberal with their interpretation and narrowed the definition down to "human being who is on your side". History is riddled with wars fought in blasphemous uses of Gods name.

Islam, supposedly the fastest-growing religion on the planet[123], quotes several times in its Koran, that one should show respect for animals:

.but to hunt. is forbidden you, so long as ye are on the pilgrimage. Be mindful of your duty to Allah, unto Whom you will all be gathered. (Koran, surah 5, verse 96)

> Then God said, "I give you every seed-bearing plant on the face of the whole earth and every tree that has fruit with seed in it. They will be yours for food." - Genesis 1:29

The teaching states, in Mecca, the birthplace of Mohammed, no creature can be slaughtered and that perfect harmony should exist between all living beings. Which is odd, as I can't quite imagine that all the restaurants there are vegan.

Whoever is kind to the creatures of God is kind to himself. (the Prophet Mohammed).

So it seems Mohammed was not always kind to himself, as he also partook in feasting on the flesh of others.

There is not an animal on the earth, nor a flying creature flying on two wings, but they are all peoples like unto you. (Koran, surah 6, verse 38)

> How does Moses make his tea? Hebrews it.

Ahimsa is an east Indian term relating to the principal of non-violence toward all life, it is an important tenet of both Hinduism and Jainism, where animals are seen as sentient beings worthy of human love and protection. Killing animals for food or any other reason is supposedly completely unthinkable to an adherent of Ahimsa, although I suspect as with other religions there are disciples who will ignore or regularly turn a blind eye toward this tenet. Violence toward animals is said to negatively affect a person's destiny and fate. The concept of karma suggests *one reaps what one sows* and adherents of Ahimsa believe the violence and misery experienced by a murdered animal will be metaphysically transferred to the flesh-eater during his own lifetime.

The Bahai Faith teaches respect for animals is just, and even encourages its followers to become vegetarian. Some will even choose to cut out all animal products and eat vegan. Admittedly, not all followers have the insight enough to equate respect for animals with diet at all, so I'm guessing fully committed vegetarians in the faith are most likely to be in the minority.

Furthermore, Abdu'l-Bahá said, *Fruits and grains [will be the foods of the future]. The time will come when meat will no longer be eaten.*

The next time those Jehovah Witnesses come knocking on the door, take a look at one of their small colourful brochures. They often have one baring a picture

> "Let me tell you something, Mark. You humans, most of you, subscribe to this policy of an eye for an eye, a life for a life, which is known throughout the universe for its stupidity. Even your Buddha and your Christ had quite a different vision, but nobody's paid much attention to them, not even the Buddhists or the Christians. You humans. Sometimes it's hard to imagine how you've made it this far."
> - Prot from the film K-Pax http://bit.ly/KPaxVid

of an idyllic setting with colourful fruit baskets and lions lying peacefully next to lambs. This they see as a future paradise, clearly portraying the Isaiah prophecies[e], of a time when carnivorism will stop, even as behaviour between other species. To me, it makes perfect sense for in order to bring about such a setting, we will all need to toe the line and change our eating habits. Apparently a fact not one of those young Jehovah Witnesses I've spoken with, has ever understood or appreciated. It's like they expect the changes to happen without changing anything!

I'm quite certain a few google searches would show similar thoughts expressed by other religions; quotes which are generally swept under the carpet by leaders, scholars and followers of each religion. The Pope, head of the catholic faith, and in this respect similar to the Dalai Lama, is a regular flesh eater, devouring gluttonously all creatures great and small landing burnt on his plate.

It appears clear to me, and I repeat myself, the core of all religions is about Non-Violence and the most non-violent of all food, thus the

---

e   Isaiah 11:6 The wolf will live with the lamb, the leopard will lie down with the goat, the calf and the lion and the yearling together; and a little child will lead them.

pinnacle of religious food, is unquestionably fruit. It has the potential to be obtained with no exploitation, killing or theft from animal or plant. No unjust imprisonment, branding, castration, torture or ear punching, mutilation tags, of voiceless innocent animals. No acre upon acre of annual mono-agriculture, reliant on heavy industry tractors and harvesters, resulting in the loss of many small animals lives and the loss of habitat of creatures of all sizes. The statistics for agricultural accidents and deaths to humans alone, annually, is quite shocking, not to mention the millions of mammals and other creatures sliced by combines, harvesters etc.

Corruption

Unfortunately, as organisations, there is no common religion which hasn't lost sight of these truths. Followers instead, lose themselves in the quagmire of dogma grown around each religion, often erroneously believing they alone are in possession of the truth and all other religions are inferior to their own. Unless you share their beliefs, you are in the wrong, possibly running the risk of eternities of brimstone and treacle. Instead of unifying humanity, and bringing more harmony and compassion into the world, religion has regularly resulted in the opposite, blatantly encouraging discord and disharmony, and generally run with an almost militaristic hierarchy.

"Wolf and Lamb shall feed together, Lion and Ox eat straw side by side, there shall be no hurt done, the Lord says no life shall be forfeit" - Isaiah: 65,25

I believe that as spiritual teachings become slowly institutionalised into religions, corruption is a consequential inevitability. They become businesses and as such, the focus shifts from the essence of the original teachings, toward more one of power and financial revenue raising gain. Of course, often cleverly so, such that the sheeple who flock to their congregations often have no idea of the corruption inherent within their particular chosen brand of religion. Some will even go to the extreme of murdering others who criticise their faith, indeed, there are probably people who will dismiss this whole book and all its ideas as nonsense, based purely on the fact they feel I may have slighted their religion.

Of course, I am not at all denying inherent truths to be found within religious teachings, nor suggesting one should not believe in that which is beyond the physical. I myself, though not altogether comfortable with the word God, have unbounded faith in the Divine,

163

the great white spirit, call it what you may. I believe there is an overall fairness in all that exists, and beyond the physical we are all eternal beings. I just do not believe any one religion has a monopoly on truth. It is somewhat the "Golden Buddha" story revisited, where the essence of religion is pure spiritual gold. All the rest is mud. The elitism, the gay discrimination, gender oppression, genital mutilation, abusive dogma, the Christmas turkeys, the halal, the ghee, the threat of eternal brimstone and treacle; all mud, and not even the glorious sort one can contentedly wallow in!

Karma

Our planet is full of laws, some of them contradictory, many of them ridiculous, many of them meant only for the masses and not for the ruling elite. Some people have found ways to successfully

> "Life will give you whatever experience is most helpful for the evolution of your consciousness. How do you know this is the experience you need? Because this is the experience you are having at the moment."- Eckhart Tolle

circumnavigate certain laws and disobey them regularly. However, beyond the loopholed laws of humans, there exists a simple, yet profound, spiritual law of cause and effect. It goes by the title of Karma and one cannot hide from it.

The way I see it, Karma is a one true universal law. It is a kind of cosmic accounting system ensuring that, despite often appearances to the contrary, there is a fairness to everything. For every cause there is an effect. For every bad deed committed, negative karma is incurred, thus increasing suffering, for every good deed, the karmic burden is lessened. I believe it is because there are so many bad deeds committed, there is so much suffering within this world.

Who gets to decide what's classified as good or bad? Some may deny such a distinction even exists, but

FIVE MINUTES IN, AND MALCOLM FINALLY REALISED HE HAD MISREAD THE SIGN

deep down our subconsciousnesses, our inner beings, our souls always know. Certainly we are generally easily, readily aware when someone commits a bad deed against us, we just have to learn to be more consciously aware, when we do likewise against others. We also need to expand our definition of *others* far beyond the limitation of our own race, gender, ethnicity and species. i.e., should someone punch us for no reason, we would judge this as a bad act. If a dog bites us, we may think the dog is behaving badly, especially if unprovoked. Even if the dog is hungry and bites with the intention of eating us, we would surely protest. Should we boot the dog for no reason, then we are the one's behaving badly. It does not matter that the dog is not human. Consider now whether we should force a pig into a life of misery and suffering, to finally murder and butcher her cadaver. Should this be considered acceptable behaviour because the intention was all along to eat the fellow? Come on, use your imagination. Use your empathy!

If you truly are capable of doing so and keep doing so, then eventually you too will come to the only logical conclusion, as I have repeated on numerous occasions in the past, fruit is the only food which is truly given, both freely and generously from the plant, which willingly bequeaths it. Every other food incurs some kind of karmic debt.

A bad deed can be anything from murder, greediness, being deceitful to others or oneself (denial), not being affectionate enough, or deliberately turning a blind eye to the plight of a calf forcibly removed from his mother, robbed of his mother's affection and milk, and slaughtered for his veal. The combinations are endless. Callous uprooting of trees. What goes around, comes around.

> Religions are a fool's errand on the Path to Enlightenment.

> "CONFORMITY is doing what everybody else is doing, regardless of what is right. MORALITY is doing what is right, regardless of what everyone else is doing." - Evette Carter

Reincarnation

But how can it be true for there to be a prevalent fairness throughout existence, when there is so much about this world which on the surface seems to be so frankly unjust? How can it be fair for one person to be born into a loving family, where all their needs and comforts are met, physically, emotionally, mentally and spiritually, where food is ever present and a safe environment provided, and yet another, in stark contrast, is born into a war torn country, surrounded by poverty, or to drug abusing parents who fail to provide even the most basic of needs, who may

165

even consciously abuse their child, physically by neglect, or in other ways?

Such scenarios are sadly all too common and can easily make one question whether this fairness I propose actually exists, or whether it is perhaps just a figment of my overzealous imagination. I believe reincarnation sheds light on this apparent dilemma.

It would be so much easier if when we pressed down the wrong button, we received an immediate reprimand. Even the slowest of us would soon learn there were consequences to pressing such buttons. Unfortunately though, the universe does not work this way. There is no time limit on the effects of deeds.

Q: What did the Buddhist monk say to the hot dog vendor?
A: "Make me one with everything"

Some responses are clear to some of us, as to why we suffer the slings and arrows of certain outrageous misfortunes. Why we endure the regular bout of "the cold", for example, may be quite blatantly obvious when seen from the clarity of eating raw. However, when trying to explain why you just cut your finger, stubbed and broke your toe, twisted your ankle, or got knocked down by a random cyclist, there appears to be a randomness involved beyond any immediately recognisable cause and effect. Even with a more heightened sense of awareness things may happen resulting in one saying "Why me, why God, why?".

The reason may not at all be apparent, but I believe whatever untoward should bechance us, there is always, always, a karmic explanation. Quite possibly not even extending from this current lifetime. On the surface this can be confusing, because generally we have no recall of our past misdeeds. However, deep down, I believe there is an awareness below one's waking conscience, and if we can only acknowledge this fairness, and understand we cannot ever truly hide from our delinquent shenanigans, this can shape our present and ultimately the future of all sentience.

"Our task must be to free ourselves by widening our compassion to embrace all life" - Albert Einstein

However, with this in mind, it is important we don't fall into the trap of thinking "oh, it's okay, what they experience is just karma, thus all is deserved". If you are part of their suffering, you are yourself incurring karma, whether or not you are in some intricately complex way also helping the universe repay another's karmic debt. We cannot justify injustice by the belief

166

that we are helping some system we will never really fully understand. Because we won't! Let the universe reap its own justice. The way to quickly settle karmic scores lies through understanding, acceptance, forgiveness and compassion. Through yearning for peace with every cell of our bodies and thus becoming a magnet for it.

Divine Faith

All we really need to be successful with Eden Fruitarianism is faith in the divine and the understanding that *harm to a part, is harm to the whole*. Without such understanding, we can soon become lost in fear, doubt and consequently fail.

Of course, I may be wrong about all of this chapter. There may be no such thing as this karma I talk of. There may be no such thing as reincarnation. There may be no such thing as the soul. The Muslims may indeed be in sole possession of the truth. Or maybe the Eckists are. Or the protestants. Or the Moonies. Or the atheists. Perhaps it is all just inexplicable random atoms obeying physical laws we will never understand and there is no right or wrong. Perhaps Douglas Adams hit the nail on the head when he humorously suggested the whole universe was sneezed out of the mouth of a giant dragon, and that we should fear the coming of the great white handkerchief.

The truth is, little of the universe makes any real sense, so we should all be forgiven for the beliefs and faiths we hold. Not wanting to be limited by the finite, the concept I have outlined above makes the most sense to me and thus it is where I chose to let my faith lie.

Circle of Compassion

Regardless of how big or small it may be, we, each and every one of us, all have a circle of compassion, it's really the magnet which keeps sentience on the world sentient.

"Until mankind extends its circle of compassion to all living things, we will never truly find peace."
- Albert Schweitzer

As the saying goes, *love makes the world go around*! If the reverse were suddenly true and none of us had a circle of compassion, sentience would soon trickle to a halt. This is about as likely to happen as it is that the world's gravitational pull to be suddenly switched off.

I find it difficult to imagine that there may be any individual being alive whose circle is limited to purely themselves. Even the most cold blooded of creatures, such as the crocodile, has a circle of compassion encompassing more than just her own unique being. If this were not the case, nothing would prevent her from eating her own eggs or newborn hatchlings. Instead the mother croc will gently carry her offspring to a place of safety and some will even care for and protect their young for up to three months until they are grown enough to care for themselves. Of course, crocodiles are hardly brimming, bubbling and overflowing with love. Far from it, their circles of compassion barely extend beyond their known family within immediate territorial range, but this still doesn't stop love being the predominant driving force keeping the species continuing.

Lions, the degenerates of the jungle, will sacrifice themselves to protect their cubs and have circles of compassion often extending to encompass the small tribes they live in. Some have even been known to adopt the young of other species, I recall one particular case from the beginning of the 21st century, where a lioness even adopted an oryx[124], a species of antelope native to Africa! Then there is the case of Little Tyke[125], another lioness, which refused point blank to eat meat!

One's circle of compassion is basically a way of describing the sphere of sentience which we care for. Even for some humans it may be just immediate family members and friends, and indifference toward the fate of anyone outside of the circle. It's likely some of this group might include individuals not of our own species. Their cat(s) and/or dog(s) for example. Others might extend their circle to include all members of their tribe or village or city, country or members of their own ethnicity, religious belief system, culture or supporters of the same football team. Many feel compassion for every other human being and are saddened by any human suffering, seeing us all as human and worthy of respect and dignity.

"Spirituality is NOT a religion. Being spiritual just means you are in touch with your own divine self." - Anna Pereira

Some, currently a minority, consciously choose to widen their circles yet further, to embrace other species beyond the narrow confines of the canines and felines and wish to avoid intentional harm to most other land animals; mammals, birds and reptiles. From there, it's but a small step to experience empathy for creatures of the oceans and waterways too and to wish them all no harm. These people understand there is no valid logical reason to exclude such creatures from their circles, especially one based purely upon their difference of appearance and or intellectual capacities and see no reason why they should be any less respectfully treated and honoured.

Some circles have grown to envelope specific plant life too. This may mean caring for a particular prized pot plant that's both caressed and softly spoken to daily. Or it could be a much loved tree at the bottom of the garden, appreciated for the shade it provides, and its intricate branches perfectly suited for climbing, or simply the delicious mulberries it gives generously each year.

Then there are those who concede that the humble carrot, in its own silent way, may be none too agreeing with being uprooted and munched on. Such a person needs no scientific proof of this, much less than he or she might need scientific proof of injustice inflicted on a goldfish confined to a small bowl, or that a canary suffers from his improper imprisonment, or that a dog is aggrieved from a sudden sharp smacking. Especially with the realisation that fruit is a viable solution to the live and let die paradigm, even if there is uncertainty of the experience of the likes of a beetroot, there can certainly be no harm in giving such life the benefit of the doubt and letting it live blessedly.

> "It is foolish to expect true happiness from earthly attachments and possessions, for they are powerless to bestow it. Yet millions of people die of broken hearts, having tried vainly to find in worldly life the fulfilment that exists only in God, the source of all joy." - Dr. M.W. Lewis

The good thing about the circle of compassion, is the lack of boundaries. One can forever keep extending the outer limits. Looking beyond the mistreatment and abuse of animals inherent throughout most of society as we know it, we can see the destructive effect our presence has on the environment and the rest of nature and do our darnedest to try and minimise it.

In defence of keeping the circle tight, people will often argue, that you can't possibly ever encompass everything and thus conclude the pointless of even trying. But this argument is so irrelevant. Even if there are compromises and things still "get hurt", this would be no reason for us to not make efforts and grow through doing so. It does not make us hypocrites if we acknowledge there are times when our presence is unavoidably linked with the hurt of others. As we grow, we can surely

> "Forces of light on earth shall overcome the forces of darkness. Complete spiritual enlightenment on earth will occur." - Edgar Cayce

169

learn to avoid such situations.

Tikkun Olam

I came across an interesting concept recently, something known as Tikkun Olam[126], it's a Hebrew phrase which can be translated as "healing and restoring the world". It suggests humanity shares responsibility (with the Divine creator) to heal repair and transform the world. This is somewhat connected to the biblical fall from grace and implies things aren't quite as they should be and so we as humans are partially responsible, if not for the fall, then at least for restoring the splendour of the pre-fall epoch.

The Long and the Short of it.

> "Love and compassion are necessities, not luxuries. Without them nothing can survive." - Dalai Lama

Hopefully, these examples can demonstrate that Eden Fruitarians are liberationists, and not somehow religious fundamentalists. Really it matters little what your own personal beliefs are concerning any divine deity, guardian angels or potential afterlife, or if you should choose to believe so, lack of any. Eden Fruitarianism is essentially not about religious beliefs but about an understanding of the *golden rule* and an awareness of one's *circle of compassion* and the very real need to expand it. The after life that should be our highest concern and recognised as clearly influencable, is the world we leave our children.

Eden Fruitarianism is not about forcing a personal view onto anyone. It is about open mindedly recognising consciousness and questioning any variety of exploitation or violence toward any form of sentience. To compare it to religion is to fail to grasp the difference between faith and a moral argument. It's the equivalent of comparing human rights to a belief in the love Goddess Ishtar.

> "Avoiding harm to all creatures, this is true knowledge, all the rest is ignorance." Bhagavad Gita

Actually, I was pleased to read this morning, the new pope, Pope Francis, unlike his conservative predecessors, stated that salvation is there for all regardless of religious faith, atheists too and is to be obtained through good behaviour, not through belief in Christ (as has been the prior Christian axiom)[127].

SECTION THREE

THE VISION

WELCOME
to PARADISE.
365 DAYS OF PERFECT WEATHER

NO LOCKS, NO CRIME, NO THREATS, NO WORRIES!

"Non-violence leads to the highest ethics,
which is the goal of all evolution.
Until we stop harming
all other living beings,
we are still savages."
- Thomas Edison

"Why fit in, when you were born to stand out?"
- Dr. Seuss

NATURE

Up until this point, I believe there is a rudimentary truth surrounding every issue raised so far, and anyone serious enough, who can put aside old prejudices and society brainwashing, and give more thought to these things, will understand there is a very real need for change. For sure, many will not find themselves prepared enough to embrace every notion I've aired, but the essence of each chapter's message is I believe indisputable. (Go ahead, feel free to try!).

This chapter introduces a future vision, a scenario which I suppose will likely, currently, only be embraced by the few. It is, I believe, a vision of positive change and whether or not you are willing to share it with me, deters me not from pursuing it. Be prepared for something different.

> If a man cold bloodedly kills another, society might judge him to be evil and incarcerate him. However if he were to murder and then eat his victim, we'd likely consider him quite sick and in need of psychiatric treatment. - Welcome to the jungle.

The Food Chain

Even those who reside in cities, with little contact with nature's wilderness, will surely be aware, through the miracle of TV and the likes of David Attenborough, that life on earth is rarely anything but peaceful.

Turn on any nature show and the dog eat dog world we live in, will be overwhelmingly apparent. Some of us feel discomfort when the crocodile jaw's clamp themselves onto the rump of a passing wilder-beast, yet it's a rare individual who will actually question whether or not this *live and let die* path is the only possible scenario for this world. Indeed, most people would argue that in order for any life to continue its existence, other life must inevitably be sacrificed. That it's just a sad fact of life, whether it be through the flesh eating of another animal or the untimely death of plant life, violence of some form is unavoidable.

> "Real peace comes from enlightenment and educating people to behave more in a divine manner."
> - Carlos Santana

Challenging the Paradigm

Have you ever paused to consider whether this really need be the case; is there perhaps some other way for life to continue? I have at times broached this issue with others, so am already aware that there will be a certain percentage of the population who will be shocked to hear me question the validity of the prevailing balance of nature. Some may immediately jump to the conclusion that something must surely be wrong with me to even question whether or not things need to be the way they are, perhaps even concluding that I am not only unrealistic in questioning it, but also in some fashion proposing some form of disequilibrium, or mass extermination of certain species.

However, for me, everything I envision throughout this book is well within the realms of the *ultimately* achievable. I am certainly not proposing any physical intervention or eradication of species I deem to be unruly. Far from it. I am totally aware of how things are, and not the least bit in denial how live and let die *is* the current way of the world. However, within the expansiveness of an apparently infinite universe, I am convinced "balances of nature" can be achieved by less violent means, and despite how the situation currently is, things can and will change. Change too, is an inevitable fact of life.

> It's not about being in opposition to death, that would just be plain silly, I understand we all must leave our corporal forms. It is about opposing violence that causes that to happen prematurely. Death and murder are two very distinct things.

It seems to me, if one is forced to take the life of another, in order for oneself to continue living, then such an existence is a very cruel, unloving, inconsiderate, malevolent, uncaring, contemptible, ungodly way of being. I suspect things may not always have been this way, and at some point in the likely distant past, there may have been some kind of, for want of a better term, biblical fall from grace, rendering the world on its current path of chaotic disrepair.

However, whether or not such a fall ever took place, is not really the issue in question. The way I see things, is quite logical and can be viewed and understood by anyone prepared to invest some moments of contemplation on the following:

If someone attempts to harm me, with no apparent cause or provocation, I will naturally protest and attempt to safeguard myself against injury. Whether it be by fleeing the scene, attempting to appease said person through words, or through otherwise defending myself in some fashion, is irrelevant. Regardless of whether such an onslaught should succeed in harming me, I will likely rule such an act as being unjust. If someone does likewise with yourself, I will undoubtedly reach the same conclusion of judgement. I find it quite probable that you too will reach the same conclusion given such hypothetical circumstances. No one deserves to be attacked without cause.

Now, if I am walking through the forest, minding my own business and a bear happens to cross my path and attempts to attack me, I will still pursue the same course of action (short, perhaps, of trying to verbally reason with the old chap) and do my utmost to avoid being harmed. The fact it's a bear I'm threatened by, and not a fellow human, will make little difference toward my feelings of danger/threat and the instinctive need of self preservation. The protagonist's species will make little difference to my feelings of the whole attack being unjust. Sure you can reason that I was on her territory, or that she was hungry, but my personal safekeeping will come first, and whether or not the bear is hungry I would still not willingly offer myself up as food, nor feel like my furry sister should be physically attacking me, when I know myself I am of absolute zero threat to her, or her potential cubs. I would equally feel empathy and concern for anyone who happened upon a bear in a forest and regardless of what's going on in the bear's mind, or tummy, still not be happy with the bear's behaviour.

> "There is only one way to avoid criticism - do nothing, say nothing and be nothing." - Aristotle

Of course, at this point in the plot, you are likely thinking, "but what about the hunger of the bear?". Isn't it odd, now that the assailant is non-human, how we immediately start preparing a verbal defence for the offender. Like suddenly because the aggressor's shape, form and DNA is slightly different to our own, this somehow justifies their action? If we were talking of a human aggressor here, living out on the moors, catching the occasional backpacker, then murdering and eating them, we would be horrified. I mean, it's one thing to kill someone, but completely something else to then bloodily butcher and devour the corpse!

And you still insist the bear is hungry, she doesn't know any better, she feels threatened, and behaves in the only way she knows how; Instinctively. Well, let us put aside the bear for a moment. The first thing needed is empathy for the victim, the hapless fellow who innocently minding his own business, stumbles into the wrong place, at the wrong time. Can we at least agree, none of us desire to take on that role? And for very valid reasons! Now instead of a bear, substitute a lion and instead of a human, a guileless gazelle which grazes his way into the picture. Is it not too gargantuan a task to feel the gazelle is also being unjustly treated?

Is it really of consequence who is doing the victimising and who is being victimised? Sympathy should be *predominantly* with the victim. Predominantly, because it is easier to feel compassion for the victim, but, agreed, sympathy and compassion are naturally ultimately for us all, regardless of our habits. To repeat, it matters little to me who the victimiser might be. What shape and form he, she or it may currently be manifested in. If they are inflicting sufferance upon others, then something is not quite as it ultimately should be. For it seems to me, once we have judged flesh eating to be ungodly, then there is little reason in not understanding this to its full conclusion. Something perhaps only a few vegans have given thought to!

One cannot be oblivious to the dilemma of the appetite of the predator though. Lions and tigers and bears (oh my!) have to eat too. Just I'd rather it wasn't me and although I likely don't know you, I'd still rather it wasn't you too, nor any other living sentient being. So what should they eat, when they have such sharp claws and razor sharp teeth, so clearly designed for occasionally ripping flesh asunder? A vision of Eden posits they can change, they can evolve into more peaceful creatures, capable of living in harmony with their entourage. Not only can they change, but when humans finally stop idolising such species as model earthlings, when we stop looking up to them as examples of how we ourselves should live, eat and behave, and begin instead to be truly civil, conducting ourselves more compassionately (thus setting ourselves as shining examples to follow), that such a change will be inevitable. And if, for whatever reasons, they are ultimately incapable of evolving toward the light side, then they will likely go the way of the dodosaurs, and abandon our earthly plains.

> Harm to a part, is harm to the whole.

Transcendental Experiment

An event that took place in the 1990s; a global political party with a spiritual agenda calling themselves "the natural law party", declared they could lower the crime rate of a city through the group practice of transcendental meditation[128]. Several demonstrations of this were undertaken, both in the US and the UK, as well as other countries, apparently with varying degrees of success[129]. I mention this solely as substantiation and evidence, of how the power of positive thought can have beneficial effects on the surrounding masses without anyone necessarily being aware of the transmission of those meditative cerebrations.

I'm not suggesting we all sit down and meditate on converting the hyenas, although clearly such an action would not be detrimental on any level. What is suggested though, is for we humans, in many ways a pinnacle species on this planet, to change our own ways, to become more harmonic. Merely by doing so, other species will be influenced likewise. The reverse has been shown to also be true. Chimpanzees living in reasonably close proximity of humans, have learned to hunt down prey, whereas genetically similar bonobos living away from the sphere of human influence, survive without the need to hunt and kill their supper.

> "Energy flows where attention goes."
> - Hawaiian Proverb

One Thousand Monkeys

You've probably all heard of the 'thousand monkeys' story? No, it's not the one where they sit down and collectively compile the complete works of Shakespeare! It goes like this: There's a group of islands some irrelevant place on the planet, and among other creatures on these islands, live an equally irrelevant species of monkey. Their main food source is some kind of tuber, a yam of sorts which they dig from beneath the ground. Anyhow, one day, this one unique little monkey, makes an accidental discovery, he drops his precious yam into the shallow depths of a small stream, wherein of course he immediately plunges his arm to retrieve it. After doing so, the little fellow has a realisation, his yam is no longer gritty with soil. From this day forth, he begins deliberately submerging his yams in the stream, effectively rinsing away the grit from the surface. After a while, other monkeys begin copying their buddy, until eventually the whole population of monkeys on this particular island have followed suit and every monkey there, washes their food before eating it.

> "Imagination should be used not to escape reality, but to shape reality." - Colin Wilson

Up until this point, it all seems to be within the realm of the understandable, but something inexplicable then follows. Something beyond the realms of the readily conceivable. The monkeys on the other surrounding islands of the archipelago begin also washing their yams, despite clearly being no recognisable means of communication between them. It was as if the time was right, critical mass had been reached and all the monkeys collectively learned a new skill.

Critical Mass

There is a collective conscience that extends far beyond a single species, and although each of us may only be a single monkey, or one of a small select group, ideas grow and one day, critical mass is attained. The whole of humanity will move forward, and with them other species will follow, until one day, paradise on this earth will be manifested.

> "Certain barriers do require a critical mass of action at the right time to overcome the inertia that is greater than incremental change." - David Jaber

Yes, I'm the eternal optimist. I predict no time frame, but my conviction is genuine. There will come a day when we will stop idolising the predators, the lion will no longer be the king of the jungle, eagles will no longer be seen as *majestic* birds of prey. Instead, we will see these animals for the bullies and butchers they truly are.

Of course, carnivorism is not practised solely by so called predator animals, every species has fallen, every species has a need to evolve. The jungle is not safe for anyone. Even the lions have their blood sucked by tics. There are many aspects of an Eden evolution required, before a semblance of a successful harmonious balance can be reached.

We might for example reason that without cats and their hunting habits, rodents could easily proliferate exponentially. True, exactly why all species need to accommodate to bring about a new balance of nature. Mice, in recognising the cat as no longer a threat, can cease multiplying so profusely. Of course, the re-evolving of nature may appear ludicrous, and readers may be wondering if this vision is for real, but once expressed it becomes communicable. How does the saying about revolutionary ideas go? First they will be ridiculed, then they will be violently opposed and finally they will be accepted as elementary normal thinking.

> It seems to me that if we eat other beings, because other species do so. Then we are indeed bowing to a very primitive peer pressure.

Try not to be overly concerned about how these changes can be accomplished, concentrate on changing yourself. Focus on a world without violence and you will surely be helping toward making such a beautiful dream become a reality.

Leading the Way

Risking possibly yet more ridicule, it is my belief that even when a lion takes the life of a zebra, he is at some level aware of the atrocity he is participating in. The lion (read tiger/bear/crocodile/spider etc) knows he takes lives unwillingly and each time he does so, his soul suffers from the act. I acknowledge a balance in nature, but I see it more as a chaotic dance, the dance being the balance. Instead of it being gentle and harmonious, it is violent and full of discord.

A view from the vantage of the Eden I am expressing, shows all of nature to be suffering from this discord and crying out for help. Not just the major predators, but all life, the plants too. Continuously competing and trying to outperform one another. Everything is part of the madness. All life wants the suffering to stop, it needs it to end. Deep down all sentience wants, indeed, yearns, to stop being part of this mess. But they can't. They are perplexedly stuck in a cycle, caught in a frenzied dance, a vicious one from which they are unable to break free. They desperately need guidance and for the song to change, so the dance can smooth down with it.

"Never let small minds convince you that your dreams are too big!" - Unknown

I see it as our duty, our role, to help change the song. To change our ways and stop the harm. To be the role models we were always meant to be and to realise this is precisely what is meant when the bible says mankind has been given dominion over life on earth. To be its spiritual guidance counsellor and to move it harmoniously forward. This is the essence of Eden Fruitarianism.

"Beware: Don't choose the convenient,
the comfortable, the respectable,
the socially acceptable.
Choose something that rings a bell in your heart."
- Osho

"Change your thoughts,
and you change the world "
- Norman Vincent Peale

"By believing passionately in something that still does not exist,
we create it. The non-existent is whatever we have not sufficiently desired."
- Franz Kafka

EDEN

A False Eden

Ask someone to describe how they envision Eden to be, and many will likely picture what they consider to be an idyllic setting, perhaps a boat upon a peaceful lake teaming with fish waiting to be hooked. Perhaps their ever faithful dog and plenty of rabbits to be caught. Ahh. Such peace! Seen from the point of view of the fish and rabbits however, such a setting would be far from peaceful, idyllic and heavenly.

Mankind can now take to the skies like a bird. Like a whale, he has learned to move deep beneath the ocean and like subterranean animals, he can move under the earth. Now he just has to learn to walk upon the earth like a human.

Peace for Everyone

However, an earthly Eden, a hypothetical future earth scenario, would be an unspoiled peaceful haven for all its inhabitants, regardless of whichever species one might happen to belong to. Every living creature will be able to walk, crawl, run and hop around freely, without fear or threat. Long grass will never harbour mischievous creatures waiting opportunistically for unsuspecting victims to sink their potentially venomous fangs into.

Fangs, claws, talons and razor sharp beaks designed specifically to rip living flesh asunder will no longer be part of any creature's accessories. Creatures such as the crocodile will agree to leave their current forms behind in favour of other more harmoniously compatible vessels. Should the lions and tigers choose to join us, their bodies will transform and they will adopt new peaceful ways of being.

There will be no blood sucking vampire beings, no mosquitoes, leaches and tics, the temperature will have a year round consistency. No more seasons of barren bleak winter and snow decked landscapes. No more months of parched drought followed by monsoon rainfall and hurricanes. No more tsunamis, earthquakes and catastrophic landslides, no more floods and blight.

How can any living being ever expect to live in Eden, if they cannot behave appropriately?

If I am wrong, and there are mosquitoes, we will rejoice as they sing in our ears, content in the fact they are merely buzzing their threatless sweet love serenades.

179

Goldilocks Zone and Axial Tilt

Let's get cosmical! Astronomically speaking, the Earth is well positioned to make the dream of an Eden utopia become a reality (as I believe it once may well have been). We are already nestled snugly within the planetary Goldilocks Zone[130], the astrobiological region, neither too close, nor too distant from a star, that will allow for a planet to maintain liveable temperatures and conditions. If humans are able to start seeing themselves as true custodians of the planet, if they can clean up their act and begin being true spiritual role models for other species, then the only thing left, to make Eden a reality, would be for the Earth's obliquity[131] (its Axial tilt) to straighten itself up.

Although it does vary minimally, due to the influence of the moon's gravitational pull, currently, it is tilted at an angle of roughly 23 degrees. Were it to be straightened up entirely, and the angle to be reduced to a vertical 0°, there would be no more seasons. No more harsh winters or excessively hot summers. No more torrential rainy seasons, followed by months of drought. No more annual cyclone and tornado seasons. Of course, this is all supposing the Earth's forests are reinstated and that humanity and other species have their acts together.

A big ask, you might think, but for an eternal optimist, like myself, although the scenario may seem improbable, if things can ultimately be better there, let's head there! Let's not worry about things so far ahead on the path, that they bear no real consequence to the current right decisions needing taking. Trust that there will always be solutions to any problems encountered on the journey! Don't pooh-pooh the idea, we live in a universe of infinite possibilities. If you believe this is an impossible dream, don't let it deter you from still moving in that direction. If it feels right, just head in that direction.

When we are ready for Eden, it will be ready for us!

> "Imagination is the beginning of creation. You imagine what you desire, you will what you imagine and at last you create what you will." - George Bernard Shaw

Walkabout

Indigenous people of mainland Australia had this rather beautiful tradition called Walkabout[132]. When they became of age, they would step out of their comfort zone, leave the familiar and habitual, and walk out into the world on their individual quests for adventure and enlightenment. I believe many will once more recognise the beauty of this practice, and will choose also to undertake such pilgrimages. Of course, this does not mean they will be catching and smashing turtles or battling wits against a snake they wish to flay and devour. Neither does it mean they'll know which logs to check for witchetty grubs[133]. The trees will bear fruits of all kinds and abundantly, such that wherever we choose to explore, we shall always have food. There will be more varieties of fruit, with fruits more wonderful than the durian, more tantalising than the chempadeks, and more sweet and yummy than the sweetest and yummiest fruits presently on the earth today.

As we peregrinate, we will carry fruit seeds with us, plant them in appropriate places as we go, and share them with others we encounter to care for. Even when we need to urinate and defecate we will do so consciously, on and around small fruit tree seedlings, and communicate with them in the process.

> What do you call a crocodile wearing a vest? - An investigator!

We will all be able to wander naked wherever we choose and with each step we take, new wonders will become visible to us. Because the temperatures will be constant and the environment totally safe with neither fear nor threat, we will be able to lie down anywhere to sleep.

Left behind loved ones will be totally at peace with our departure. One may miss another, but will rest assured of their safety. And what a joyous day it will be when reunited and all the stories we will have to share. Remember, we take to company, that which we gather in solitude. To make Eden a reality, we must all step out of our comfort zones, and make our lives legendary!

Continuing the Vision

Fruit will be understood. We will know that while the fruit hangs from the tree, the tree is in rapture. I believe they are like bliss receptors for the tree, ravishing unquantifiable cosmic love energy into its powerful core. Each slight brush of the breeze against the fruit, is like a lover's caress. Tiny orgasmical sparks that spiral inwardly. Finally, exhausted from the experience, the tree

> "I alone cannot change society for the better. But I can radically transform my own consciousness, overturning the conditioning that limits my potential. We can all do this, one by one. Over time we can change ourselves to the degree that society changes from the inside out. Giving birth to a new way of being. Manifesting our birthright of living in a peaceful and abundant world. Have no fear. Trust yourself. Live your full potential." - Unknown

lets them go. They don't have to be forcibly cut or turbulently yanked from the tree, disturbingly terminating the tree's exhilaration. Just slight nudges and the tree will bequeath its fruit to us. Don't forget, the tree wants for you to share in the bliss! Pleasures shared, are pleasures doubled!

Because of the non-existent axial tilt, even the extreme poles of the planet, barring of course any precious clean waters for our aquatic brethren, will be of constant ideal temperatures, suitable for the growing of the most tropical of fruits.

"Love all creation and you will feel heaven on earth."
- Anthony Douglas Williams

The ocean's sentient life will be equally at peace, no more big fish eating little fish. No more constantly having to watch your back. Intermingling of species will be normal with no animal fearing another and no animal taking advantage of a blissful lack of fear. Because we will be in constant proximity to other life forms, the thought of capturing another and forcing him or her into a life of servitude through dominance and forced dependence, will never enter our minds. There will be no need for harnessed pets that become reliant on us for their food and comfort. This does not mean we cannot have a special animal as a true friend, but we will never have the aberrant possessive need to cage or chain her or even to neurotically agonise where she is at all times.

Have you ever noticed, while out walking in the countryside, how the sounds of insects and birds and nature are always off in the distance? Like never up close? It's like you are walking in a bubble, with nature noises pretty much always beyond a roughly fixed distance. Pretty much all creatures currently fear us. As soon as we draw near, they stop their singing. As we approach they jump, run, flee, and fly away from us. If they don't, they stand stock still in hiding. Nothing trusts us, everything goes into "danger mode" as we approach. Step toward a frog you can hear ribbiting in the foliage, and she will instantly stop.

In Eden, with the absence of such apprehensiveness, bird's will be at ease singing right in front of us. Thoughts of catching or being caught will cross no one's mind. No one will be victimised for being happy and chirpy. We'll be able to walk up and look closely at the feathers of a bird and their beautiful little faces while they sing out in blissful glee of life. If they fly off, it will be because something more exciting and mind boggling has reached their attention.

There will be streams and rivers and waterfalls to marvel and bathe in and under. Survival of the fittest and this obnoxious idea of a food chain, will be a thing of the bygone past, belonging to a dark ages, not forgotten, but *never* celebrated.

Because we no longer fear, shun and have this innate perverse desire to conquer nature, turning it from its vibrant greens and rainbow coloured flowers into the drab dull grey of concrete, we will no longer suffer boredom.

In Eden, there will be no sharp spiked plants. The roses will be thornless, the thistles too. Have you ever noticed how, after the earth has been pillaged, its trees felled and uprooted and top soil laid bare, the first plants to make a resurgence are generally thorned. Take the cactus or the brambles, which readily grow into such environments. It is as if the Earth, after having being raped and desecrated, is saying *"Don't touch me there! I'm sore! Leave me alone!"*. And yet the Earth, as Gaia the entity, knowing our true food, still bestows us with her fruit, the blackberry and the prickly pear. Because the Earth will be healed, the thistles, spines, prickles and thorns will be no longer be required.

Gaia currently suffers from our negligence. She is ashamed that one of her children takes what she freely gives, and greedily seeks material gain from it. That we, the supposed contemplative ones, barely think twice. We, the ones that should be planetary stewards, guiding the planet into ever more colour

Flowers

Nobody's hating,
everybody's loving,
let's all go and sniff flowers.

Red ones, orange ones,
long thin limy ones,
think I'll go and sniff flowers,
big fat greeny ones,
short stubby yellow ones,
sniff, sniff, sniff, sniff flowers.

Purple, on the tree,
pink and blue and free,
rainbow red, rainbow violet,
scarlet flowers,

starry ones, perky ones,
little fairy blossom ones,
fragrant little, spotty little flowers.
Delicate and fancy,
extravagantly schmancy,
fluffy little, snuffy little flowers.

So precious, so tender,
So smooth and silk and slender,
huffy little, puffy little flowers.
Dew drop covered splendour,
pollenacious vendor,
delicious little, balmy little flowers.

Hues of luminosity,
buds of preciosity,
Fresh and pink and dandy,
chocolate stripy sandy,
petal scented candy,
sniff, sniff, kiss, bliss flowers.

and freshness, instead trash everywhere we go. With awakened realizations, all this will change.

The flowers will be more appreciated, with their vibrant iridescence and intricate patterns we will all be in wonder and awe over them. Their fragrance will be ambrosial and offer sustenance for the soul.

Insects will lose their sting for we will be more aware of their presence and less likely to brush accidentally against them. The thought of stealing their hard earned food supplies will be unthinkable, and all compulsion to kamikazecally protect the hive, obsolete. No animal will carry venom. No plants will be poisonous to the touch, or burn upon contact.

Even the plants amongst themselves will have abandoned their competitive and invasive habits. No plant shall ever have parasitic tendencies. No more strangling and slowly sapping the life out of another plant.

Gentle touch is an entirely separate issue though. All life enjoys the sensation of loving touch. If we touch

> "God gave our first parents the food he designed that we should eat. It was contrary to His plan to have the life of any creature taken. There was to be no death in Eden. The fruit of the trees in the garden was the food man's wants required."
> - Ellen White, (co-founder 7th Day Adventists.).

and/or are touched by a loved one, it feels good. If we stroke an animal that loves and fully trusts us, he will feel pleasure at the touch. We both will. It matters not what species of animal, once mutual trust has been gained, both will benefit from touch. It can be mammal, reptile, bird or insect. I imagine even spiders enjoy being touched lightly without fear of threat.

Plants too, they will be in bliss from the attention directed toward them. In Eden we will all be at ease and comfort with touch. No one and no thing will be a threat, so the touching of spirits will lift us up as if by wings. And each mind we encounter will be a different hue. Like rainbow snowflakes. Minus the chill factor.

The topsoil will be an ideal thick rich humus that retains moisture, making it a perfect sprouting terrain for young fruit tree saplings, and with enough rain or morning dew to render the requirement for human irrigation null and void.

Even the voices of beings will change and adapt to the new prevailing harmoniousness, resonating better with the rest of the environment.

184

Think how currently communication of certain animals is not exactly pleasant; a barking dog can really play on one's nerves, and not in a good way! If dogs wish to continue as a species, this will change, if they wish to keep their voices, chords will be realigned. The volume of voices will change too, such that every voice will blend perfectly with the euphonious symphony of nature.

Eden is a bold statement of symbiosis. Everything done, every action, every thought, will be not only of benefit to the thinker and doer, but of benefit to all surrounding parties too. The current parasitic balance of nature will be no more.

If again, you find yourself shaking your head in disbelief, thinking without the current system of checks and balances, without the presence of the carnivores, their prey will breed proliferously, think again. It is clear the changes needed to pull this off will not be restricted solely toward carnivorous habits. Lifeforms currently falling victim to barbed, clawed and sabre fanged beasts, will no longer breed epidemically. Instead of going forth and multiplying proliferously, we shall all be at peace and living splendiferously. We will come to realise it is precisely the threat of the blood lusting carnivores that proliferous epidemic overpopulating exists in the first place!

> "When we care for every living being on earth, we will stand on heaven's ground."
> - Anthony Douglas Williams

Of course, even if there were to be a sudden global awakening, the transition to Eden would likely still not happen overnight. This will likely take time and there will first be a great upheaval and turmoil. Similar to that which is experienced while the body is being cleansed through detox, only on a much grander scale. A microcosm/macrocosm thing. The earth has been grossly abused and short of divine intervention, there must be time for healing.

There is no need to get too hung up on the complexity and scale of the changes needed, to fulfil such a vision, astronomically our lives are but brief gnats' farts in time, so if you are reading this in fifty, one hundred or two hundred years from now and things have seemingly gotten worse, hold the vision and for each one of us doing so, we bring the reality of it closer.

Any idea we might currently hold of "how boring", will be lost in the awesomeness of it all. I wonder how many people have ever walked Machu-Picchu and thought "how boring!". There are waterfalls near

185

us, I often take visitors there, not one has come away thinking "that was dull!".

Once harmonic order has superseded the current state of disharmonic chaos, the necessity for change will be self evident to all, and we will all puzzle why it took so long.

There will be no money. No more accounting. Not even bartering. The mentality of sharing will be universally adopted by all, and exchange will be no more.

It is a law of economics, that for a thing to have a price, it has to be scarce, insufficient, therefore there must be an abundance, like the air we breath, and the price has to be zero.

Royalty, landowners and governors, politicians and butchers will become "once upon a time, in a galaxy far, far away" enigmas. From the bizarre land of cabbages and kings. It may not be blatantly obvious to most of us, but plants experience indignation when they are swapped for money, trees feel belittled and humiliated when their fruits are stripped and sold. All this is given freely and joyously, and humans have brought shame and dishonour to the earth by such flagrant profiteering.

Naturally there will be no wars, nor struggles for dominance and power. How can there be when greediness is put aside for empathy. When faith replaces fear. When jealousy is replaced by plenitude and trust. There will be no more boundaries and border guards preventing us from walking freely in any direction we choose.

There will be no more patriotism, no more nationalism, no more countries and passports, no more neurotic, bullying, border guard officials, who unquestioningly follow orders deporting, detaining and imprisoning those who wish to practise their innate birthright to travel. The only law will be to do as one wishes, provided it does not intrude on the privacy, nor jeopardise the health and safety of any other living being.

"You cannot depend on your eyes when your imagination is out of focus." - Mark Twain

Any creativity channelled into devices or technology, will be done so with a full awareness of consequences, such that no life is injured or dismayed in the process, nor will there be any harmful long term ramifications of such. With the new globally evolved consciousnesses, parts of the brain will be unlocked such that much of technology we think of today as essential, will no longer be required. Telepathy may enable us to sing to one another in our minds, and to be in touch regardless of distance.

One thing for sure in the world as it currently exists; human creativity has evolved far beyond its spirituality, thus we have unlocked nature's secrets to create technology which is first and foremost, used by darker powers, for destructive purposes. Humankind's spirituality needs to catch up by leaps and bounds, keeping a check on technological innovation and intentions, such that if a new secret of the atom is unveiled, its destructive weapon potential is fully disregarded.

"There is no Wi-Fi in the forest, but I am sure you will find a better connection." - Unknown

The long and the short of it, beings are not mean to each other in Eden, there is an ampleness of everything, and nobody will try to deceive another, or trick another into deals that are not to everyone's benefit. With the complete and utter absence of struggle and strife on all levels, peace fills the void.

It is a difficult task, considering the current sad state of disrepair the world is currently lost within, but we must do our bests to behave as if such a world already exists. By doing so, we help pull it towards us. This is indeed a challenge, but really, how can we expect to ever live in Eden, if we cannot ourselves behave appropriately?

How do I know how things are in Eden? Well, quite frankly, I don't of course. I think I've made it clear already that the views expressed within this book are based on faith, not already indisputable scientific fact. Unlike most authors of similar books I am not telling you that anything I say is fact, I am not talking as if I have irrefutable knowledge. That doesn't make me any less confident and convinced of my stance and view point. And it shouldn't make my opinions any less valid. In fact most authors of diet related literature kid themselves and their readers in stating their opinion is the unquestionable truth.

A person without imagination is like a flavourless durian.

I'm not a gambling man, but if I were, I'd consider it a sound wager to bet my bottom dollar, that if you were to turn up at Eden carrying a fishing rod and/or shotgun, or even with the mere notion that some of its free ranging critters were potential food items, or there to capture, subdue and ride, or that living trees were perfect for felling, I expect you'd be politely but firmly told to move along, and take your business elsewhere. If you don't like the vision I'm sharing, then find another one, or make up your own!

187

Paradise Restored

For the biblically orientated, there are some quite beautiful passages affirming such a vision as an eventual outcome. Parts of Isaiah are worth pointing out once more: "The wolf will live with the lamb, the leopard will lie down with the goat, the calf and the lion and the yearling together." (Isaiah 11:6) and "The wolf and the lamb will feed together and the lion will eat straw like the ox; but as for the serpent, its food will be dust! They won't harm or destroy on my entire holy mountain," (Isaiah 65:25).

> "It is part of the destiny of the human race, in its gradual improvement, to leave off eating animals, as surely as the savage tribes have left off eating each other"- Henry David Thoreau

Also, Matthew 6:25 and onward is particularly relevant. It's basically to remind us we should have more faith. We should look at the birds of the air and realise how without all the sweat and toil humans are fond of, all their needs are still met. It's true, it seems like most animal species have their place on earth, (albeit not without issues) and all their basic needs, not counting free from threat, are met. Humans though, really seem to be an exception to the rule. Take society away from even the most able people and they will struggle to survive. Is the reason for this because our ideal environment no longer exists on this planet? Eden is where we ultimately belong. The environment we are most well suited for. It may have been here once already, but if it has, it's clearly been trashed.

*How can any of us ever expect to live in Eden
if we cannot act accordingly?*

*"I am going to venture that the man who sat
on the ground in his tipi meditating on life,
and its meaning, accepting the kinship of all creatures,
and acknowledging unity with the universe of things
was infusing into his being the true essence of civilization."*
- Luther Standing Bear,
(Oglala Lakota Sioux (1868-1939))

THE EDEN FRUITARIAN

At time of writing, the Eden Fruitarian is an extremely rare individual, a pioneer moving against the grain, however, there will come a day, when everyone on the planet will be one.

The Eden Fruitarian understands the basic principles outlined in the previous chapters, and knows that these concepts will one day inevitably be understood and embraced by all life. He, (and I mean that in the most genderless of ways), is realistic about these changes, and understands that first and foremost, we must become the change we wish and need to see.

It's a challenge few are currently genuinely willing and ready to face up to, and even fewer have the will power, faith and conviction to succeed. Understandably so, as it's not as if the world we live in makes

189

things easy. All around us we are surrounded by temptation, obstacles, negativity and opposition. The vast bulk of us have an awful lot of emotional baggage and dependency on those temptations and obstacles. Eden Fruitarianism goes against most of what we have been taught, so it's inevitable that when aired publicly, one should expect it to be ridiculed and criticised.

Well meaning family and friends will likely do their utmost, to stop you pursuing such a path. Perhaps, and I'm musing here, it is because deep down they fear to be left behind. But it is precisely fear which the Eden Fruitarian needs to forsake.

> "The most fundamental moral obligation and responsibility of humanity is to protect and preserve our divinely manifested, and therefore sacred, garden planet, Earth and all life on it; maintaining it all in near pristine condition. We are God's gardeners!" - Matali

There comes a time in everyone's life, when we must stand on our own two feet, and choose our own direction and path. This is of course a metaphorical path, and does not necessarily mean one has to break contact with those one loves and is loved by. It does however mean one has to learn to stand one's ground, and be prepared to move against the current of social norms.

Although, as history has shown, some have made headway, changing the entire world, by any one person alone, is a gargantuan task. What is well within the realm of the feasible, is for us each to change and shape our own small worlds and environments. We must seek to make our environment as Eden compatible as we can, to facilitate our path and direction of focus. For many, this may mean being brave and leaving behind the ease of the familiar and seeking out a new home more fitting to one's needs. Likely this will require faith, but that's a good thing, for each time we rely on faith, we are bound less and less to fear.

> "Many People, especially ignorant people, want to punish you for speaking the truth, for being correct, for being you. Never apologise for being correct, for being years ahead of your time. If you're right and you know it, speak your mind. Even if you are a minority of one, the truth is still the truth." - Gandhi

Given that the world is as it is, certain behavioural facets of Eden Fruitarianism may not immediately be practical, but this should not stop us focusing on other achievable aspects, nor should we fall into the trap of using those tricky details as excuses to hold us back, from following other qualities more readily obtainable and doable.

Firstly, as budding Eden Fruitarians, it is our duty to bring our diets more into accord with Eden principles. This involves eating as high on the ethical food tower (outlined in the Eden Fruitarianism chapter) as we are able. We should, realise that animals are neither there to satisfy our gluttony, nor to sadistically imprison for testing purposes, nor to butcher as potential clothing items, nor to imprison as visual entertainment in zoos and circuses nor as household company, nor to be part of any other industry reliant on their captivity and abuse.

"The miracle of your mind isn't that you can see the world as it is. It's that you can see the world as it isn't." - Kathryn Schulz

He does his best to avoid all unnecessary chemicals, whether they be on our foods, or as household cleaning products. Fruit has cleansing properties both externally as well as internally. It feels great to massage mango or papaya peal into one's skin and then jump into a fresh water stream! Or lemon juice can be a great substitute for shampoo, especially when one first begins to break free from the regular shampooing most of us grow accustomed to. A daily rinse in water is all one ultimately needs to keep the hair clean and head itch free.

The Eden Fruitarian recognises the body as the temporary sacred temple of the soul. He (again the implied genderless pronoun) understands it is our duty to keep it internally clean and clutter free. Among other things, this will better help us to appreciate the resounding universal hum of OM. We have far more responsibility toward our body than the owner of an expensive piece of machinery needing safeguarding, regular adjustment and high quality fuel. He understands fruit to be the highest quality fuel, most well suited for human physiology, and will go out of his way to ensure such fuel is always steadily, readily available. He understands that wine is not fruit juice and that all alcoholic beverages should be avoided, even in small irregularly taken quantities. Equally, other mind altering substances are shunned, in favour of the

No one can drive you crazy unless you give them the keys!

euphoria to be had from the intricate fragrance, taste and texture, of the likes of durian and other exotic fruits, that are mere fractions of what will come to be.

191

Externally the body is ours to protect and watch over too, and this does not mean we should territorially carve our initials onto it with tattoos, nor punch holes through it as piercings. Neither does it mean we should regularly paint graffiti over it, in the form of make-up. The idea of plastic surgery, to somehow enhance the body's form, is also clearly seen as a ludicrous, sacrilegious concept which sadly too many of today's earthlings with apparently low self esteem feel drawn toward.

> My beard grows to my toes,
> I never wears no clothes,
> I wraps my hair,
> around my bare,
> And down the road I goes.
> - Shel Silverstein

Anyone can embrace Eden Fruitarianism at any stage of their life though, so don't despair. Just because you may have made mistakes in the past, does not mean that you cannot move forward, regardless of previous ignorances, blunders and slip-ups. Can anyone here truthfully say their behaviour is totally compatible with Eden, and that they live according to all its terms and conditions? Many of us though, may surely sorely love to be given the chance in a genuine Eden. So, don't be overly discouraged by the difficulties, realise the forever giving universe is ever forgiving, and above all, it is up to ourselves to forgive ourselves, and to move on with optimism. We should laugh at our mistakes and see them as important lessons, and try our darnedest to not make the same ones again. Even if we keep failing!

The Eden Fruitarian strives to leave the cities and towns behind, and is instead naturally attracted toward more scenic settings, where naturism and sun worshipping can be practised. Naturally, by "sun worshipping" I am referring to the practice of enjoying the sun's radiant energy soaking into every pore of one's body. The Eden Fruitarian knows fresh air, sunlight and clean water are important foods for the soul, and enjoys all three at every available opportunity.

Instead of taming our head and facial hair growth to conform to a society so clearly in need of healing, Eden Fruitarians are happy to let their hair grow, regardless of gender, and the folly of forever fighting back the beard is regarded with bafflement.

> "The further a society drifts from the truth, the more it will hate those that speak it." - George Orwell

Being aware our food is rarely of the quality it should be, the Eden Fruitarian sees the importance of growing as much of one's own food as possible. He is not the slightest bit shy nor afraid of getting his hands soiled in the earth, as

192

seeds and seedlings are planted and transplanted.

The Eden Fruitarian abandons all footwear in preference to baring one's feet to the elements. He recognises the harmful affects of a long term shoe fetish, and loves the feel of regaining contact with the earth and the notion of permanent foot-zone therapy.

The Eden Fruitarian is not at all concerned with calories, carbohydrates and colostrum. He doesn't fret over vitamins, minerals and proteins, or question whether or not tomatoes should be eaten, because of a vague rumour they contain nicotine. He doesn't call fruit "sugar" and label avocado as "fat" leading to an artificially restricted intake of either. He doesn't look up to someone else for advice on what, or when and how much he should eat. He has an intrinsic understanding of the guidelines needed with concern to eating (outlined in the Eden Fruitarianism chapter) and embraces the simplicity of it all.

End the wars. Tax the rich. It's a no brainer.

The Eden Fruitarian doesn't need a cooker nor microwave, nor a cacophony of pots, pans and baking trays. He understands the difference between store bought cartoned juice, and genuine fresh juice, just as much as he gets the difference between a shrivelled prune and a plum. He generates very little in the way of rubbish, and most, if not all, of what passes through his hands, is able to be composted or recycled in some fashion.

He understands the sometimes overwhelming, finiteness of life, and that all things come to an end, and does his best to not be overly attached to material objects. He understands that we are more than just our bodies, and that there is a great white spirit, the divine, through which we are all intricately interconnected. That all life is fundamentally one, and that harm to a part, is harm to the whole.

Remember, only those who risk going too far, can truly discover how far they can go.

The Eden Fruitarian doesn't go running to the doctors at the first sign of discomfort. He has an understanding of health far exceeding that of the corner store general practitioner, and doesn't need someone to sell him drugs to suppress uncomfortable self inflicted symptoms, or to diagnose the obvious.

He doesn't smear chemical concoctions all over his skin before moving into the sunshine, and he doesn't confusedly label coconuts, sugar cane juice, and similar, as fruit.

He trusts that the path to freedom lies not through science, but through faith. In fact, he sees we all rely on faith. He places his faith in the Divine, rather than science. This ultimately gives far more peace of mind, as instead of being fundamentally in denial and under the impression that we actually know things we really don't, it requires admitting one's faith and surrendering oneself to it.

He understands if a law is unjust, it is our moral obligation to disobey it, provided we can do so without jeopardising our own safety or the safety or well-being of other living entities. An "unjust" law encompasses all that which has no real value in the eyes of Divine.

Between individual beings, as between nations,
peace means respect for the rights of others.

"Currently humanity and planet Earth
is hurtling towards unspeakable catharsis,
for this is the future that we are now creating.
.. humanity must decide whether to keep on going
down the same road to global human
and environmental obliteration or change course...
Human beings do not like change, but change we must.
Currently humanity is manifesting dystopia
(the opposite to paradise).
With a united future vision, humanity can easily
re-manifest a global paradise and a truly beautiful future for all.
This is the decision that we must all make
for we are all responsible and accountable.
The dawning of The Era of Great Change is upon us"
- Matali

"Imagine all the people living life in peace.
You may say I'm a dreamer, but I'm not the only one.
I hope someday you'll join us and the world will be as one."
- John Lennon

A BRIEF SUMMARY SO FAR

My feeling is that there are plenty of books on vegetarianism and veganism already written far more eloquently than I am capable. There are more books too, on the benefits of eating raw and predominantly fruit, all of which have their merits and explain in far more detail than I am attempting to, most of which wield whatever science there is, to back up their claims. The fundamental difference between this book and others *is* the vision I've just shared.

> "What we are doing here is part of a profound transformation that is taking place in the collective consciousness of the planet and beyond: The awakening of consciousness from the dream of matter, form and separation." - Eckhart Tolle

I believe Eden Fruitarianism goes beyond what others have priorly literally expressed and likely will challenge most readers in some way. I am happy for that.

I want to challenge. I want to make you question things you have never questioned before. I want for the shod omnivores who read the first chapters, to have "aha!" experiences, and to see the need for change. I want the vegetarian to realise that vegetarianism is not enough. I want the vegan to see the sense in ceasing to fire up food before consumption. I want for the vegan who recognises violence as abhorrent, to question whether nature's current way should be admired, just plain ignored, or envisioned differently. If one thinks that the human race would be better off without violence toward other humans or other animals, why should we not draw the next logical conclusion and question violence within nature? If one thinks violence should be intervened and prevented within the realms of human activity, should we not also begin to debate and challenge violence amongst species other than human too?

I want the raw fooders and the budding fruitarians to understand fruit from more than just a dietary perspective. For everyone to see the potential it has beyond its rudimentary undervalued status as snack food. I want for everyone to see the pet trade as a flagrantly depraved business, without any animal's welfare as its ultimate goal. I want for the shodarians to take their shoes off, to feel the earth and wriggle their toes! I want for clothing to be put under the spotlight and questioned. I want for people to open up their bathroom cabinets, and question every item they see there.

All of these desires are not based on whimsical wishes alone. There are good solid reasons to support such changes. Once you begin to question all this, with an open mind, including the current paradigm of nature's balance, the vision of Eden can become so much more than just a hopeless romantic fantasy. Even if you believe the vision will accomplish nothing, at least acknowledge that it's a beautiful one, which can do no harm!.

What would be sad, is if someone were to begin reading this book and think "Hey, there's a sense to this empathy lark", but then, when they get to the envisioning, which they are not prepared to share, they short-sightedly choose to dismiss everything else based purely on that.

> "Unless you try to do something beyond what you have already mastered you will never grow."
> - Ralph Waldo Emerson

There will indubitably also be readers who will immediately dismiss the mere idea of nature's balance changing, deeming the notion to be preposterously impossible, and yet still they will want to voice indignation that I am threatening their world as if I have a very real chance of challenging the status quo. They will protest the thought of their winters being removed, claiming that to be their favourite time of year.

I acknowledge the enjoyment some may reap from winter sports, and can myself idolise the picture of a romantic log fire in a warm and cosy log cabin surrounded by snow bedecked pine trees. Or a hot sauna followed by a quick roll in the fluffy white stuff. No denying the fun in that!

> "You have to understand, most people are not ready to be unplugged. And many of them are so inert, so hopelessly dependent on the system that they will fight to protect it." - Morpheus (The Matrix)

For the world to move forward though, especially toward Eden, we must let go of such attachments in favour of more harmonious ones. When we free our imaginations, there will be things far more awesome to witness, share and participate in!

Reap what you can from these pages. If they can assist you to stop eating flesh, to cut out dairy, to cease cooking, go for it. Don't be deterred by views beyond those you are currently able to agree with! Every step in the right direction will help bring more harmony into the world.

SECTION FOUR

VARIOUS OTHER THOUGHTS

*"Before our white brothers arrived
to make us civilised men,
we didn't have any kind of prison.
Because of this, we had no delinquents
Without a prison, there can be no delinquents.
We had no locks nor keys and therefore
among us there were no thieves.
When someone was so poor that
he couldn't afford a horse, a tent or a blanket,
he would, in that case, receive it all as a gift.
We were too uncivilized to give great
importance to private property.
We didn't know any kind of money
and consequently, the value of a human being
was not determined by his wealth.
We had no written laws laid down,
no lawyers, no politicians,
therefore we were not able
to cheat and swindle one another.
We were really in bad shape
before the white men arrived
and I don't know how to explain
how we were able to manage
without these fundamental things that
(so they tell us) are so necessary for a civilised society."*
- John (Fire) Lame Deer

FOOD SUPPLY

It is true, that in the highly hypothetical, equally improbable, situation where the world should suddenly wake up and demand more fruit, there would not be enough. Or not enough infrastructure to cope with such a sudden increase in demand. But, well, so what? This is not something anyone need be concerned about.

Eden Fruitarianism is in its infancy. There are a few pioneers, but mostly the world is completely oblivious to the philosophy. It's like a flower having its roots in

> The Mallard Drake dunks his head,
> and thick little streams,
> that look like mercury,
> go gliding down his oily back.
> While all around him,
> there are stars in the water,
> where the raindrops fall.

vegetarianism growing, from the dirt and compost of a chaotic shod omnivore world. It pushed up into veganism, then raw veganism and fruitarianism and finally Eden Fruitarianism, like a lotus flower reaching for the sky. Its bud can barely be said to be forming but will one day blossom so openly, everyone will be enraptured by its fragrance and essence.

Meanwhile, as things move around to accommodate this new concept, it is up to those of us who understand and embrace it, to help manifest more supply for those yet to follow. This can be done from wherever we are, merely by making our desires and demands more public. By growing more of our own food, or starting our own fruit supply, delivering to others who are interested, and you can be sure there will be. There are all kinds of people waiting out there in the woodwork, beginning to awaken but needing help and encouragement to do so. So if you are living in an area where there is not enough supply, don't just complain about it, if you are not prepared to move somewhere else, then do something about the lack. Make it happen! Make your needs known to the universe, and they will move toward you.

> "I don't want to protect the environment. I want to create a world where the environment doesn't need protecting!" - Unknown

Meanwhile, it is unfortunate that probably none, or very, very little at most, (yes, you read that right) of the fruit, and commercially available food, is fully compatible with the Eden Fruitarian philosophy. Most will have been subjected to some form of toxic chemical abuse, or other non-ethical processes, including human exploitation and genetic modification.

The most widely available alternatives of organic produce are often almost equally despicable, with heavy reliance on mammal blood and bone, or crushed fish paste sprays, as the basis for fertiliser. Fruit trees also, both conventional and organic are regularly and systematically pruned causing much destruction in the process. More on this shortly. It stands to reason that these methods are far from ideal, and should not even be considered vegan! While these often seem to be the only available alternatives, and until we explore new forms of more harmonious agriculture, whatever we choose, will in some way be a compromise.

> "The universe is full of magical things patiently waiting for our wits to grow sharper." - Eden Phillpotts

Vegaculture

Likely we've all heard of permaculture? Though the idea itself was only christened in 1978, (derived from PERManent and agriCULTURE[134]), its principle tenet being the support of people and the environment, its basic guidelines have been used, by an increasing minority throughout all cultures and eras. Take the time to read up about it and you will surely not fail to see its many advantages and truths. Since first hearing of permaculture in the 1980s, the idea has held its fascination with me, however, there is one aspect of it which has long troubled me and caused me to question its ideals; their reliance on the exploitation of animals.

This is where Vegaculture[135] comes to play, coined by my good friend Zalan Glen, it is permaculture with the added magical ingredient of Animal Empathy. VEGAn-permaCULTURE. Basically growing one's food without the use of either chemicals, or reliance on the excrement and carcasses of animals kept solely for exploitative purposes. Thus the guiding principle is one of support of people, *animals* and the environment.

Don't jump to a false conclusion and think animals are absent, chased out or discouraged from being in a Vegaculture garden though, far from it. The aim of vegaculture is not only to produce ethical clean food, but also to do so in an empathetic way, mirroring nature's diversity, thus encouraging and assisting local fauna in finding a home within your garden. It does not involve restricting their movements, stealing their eggs or violently and forcibly removing another's offspring so we may drink their milk.

The trouble with the controlled inclusion of animals within one's garden and food production, lies more than with the obvious exploitation of said animals. Granted such small scale scenarios are far more ecologically viable than modern factory farming techniques and avoid vast amounts of animal suffering, but they are still part of the problem, not the solution. Modern day factory farming has been extended from this traditional base, so in a way, permaculture is a sort of step backwards, with the question of exploitation not fully being addressed. Disregarding sentience, one might easily choose to step forward into factory farming again. VegaCulture is a true step forward, by including the welfare and freedom of animals in the design process, we can put an end to blatant disregard of animal lives.

> "There's a reason we take our kids to pick apples, but don't take them to a slaughterhouse. - Make the Connection!" - Unknown

Fruit Trees

The value of trees to the environment can never be overestimated. Many may see them solely for their potential value as timber, or for the real estate value of the land they flourish on, but they furnish so much more of what we need to survive. As well as providing air/oxygen, water and food, trees prevent accelerated soil erosion, maintain temperature by reducing the intensity of the sunshine, and by stopping heat and water evaporation from the top soil, slowing down the winds and encouraging worms.

With climate change becoming a major consideration, planting more trees is essential as they are obviously one of nature's primary and most rapid carbon storage methods.

They may take longer to begin yielding, but fruit trees provide more food per square meter of ground than any other food on this planet, with potentially much less labour involved in the cultivation and harvesting. Not only do they produce the most food, but they require far less labour, and far less soil invasion, than the production of any other food. The turning of the soil carries many deaths in its wake; both animal and plant life fall victim of the process.

The insanity of the world has seeped into all spheres, and fruit production is certainly not without its troubles. Over time, we need to all get involved at some level with primary industry, and help guide and steer it away from its harmful monocrop tendencies, and general heavy reliance on chemical unsustainability. We could begin by getting all streets lined with fruit trees, making fruit freely available for all.

I read recently of a Seattle project[136] to create a new, seven acre city park, filled entirely with all kinds of fruit trees and more. The plan is for the park to be open to anyone and everyone, to come and go as they please, and for anyone to eat freely from the garden. Such a great project! If successful it will be the first such public food forest in the US. Who knows, maybe if it is fortuitous, it will be the first of many, sparking other cities to do likewise. This kind of project needs to be implemented all around the globe.

Tree Pruning

> "The ultimate goal of farming is not the growing of crops, but the cultivation and perfection of human beings."
> - Masanobu Fukuoka

For modern day commercial fruit growers, pruning is generally a vicious and violent affair. Deafening, lumbering, crunchy contraptions wreak havoc through the orchard, compacting the soil unduly, while their indestructible, fast flying blades annihilate anything in their path. Nests, eggs and chicks go flying, as do any other unfortunate tree dwelling animals. All in order to unnaturally shape the tree, convenient for later harvest. This regular process is just as proliferous in nonorganic as organic orchards.

Lasting powerful truly symbiotic relationships can never be formed with a tree when one person (or a small team) put themselves in charge of thousands of trees. Even hundreds are too many. Yet another reason why more people need to return to primary industry and begin cultivating and growing their own fruit food.

> "We must protect the forest for our children, grandchildren and children yet to be born. We must protect the forests for those who can't speak for themselves such as the birds, animals, fish and trees."
> - Qwatsinas, Nuxalk Nation

I'd like to mention Masanobu Fukuoka, author of the book which partially inspired the permaculture movement[137]. One little story he mentioned within that book, was how as a child he had always questioned how his father would annually prune the orange trees in their orange orchard. Masanobu couldn't understand why it was necessary, and his father explained that if one didn't do so, the tree would not fruit. Later in life, after his father passed away, and he had inherited that orchard, he decided to put this theory to the test, and stopped the annual prune. Sure enough it only took a year or two, to see the orange yield plummet, just as his father had correctly predicted.

Instead though, of starting pruning once more, Masanobu decided to continue his experiment. Over the years, the branches of those trees became convoluted and tangled, and through his experimenting, many of the trees died. However, still not fully understanding why so much work was involved annually, he pushed on, this time, experimenting with new trees that never got pruned at all. The result was that they initially took longer to begin fruiting, but once they did so, the trees were giving as much, or more fruit, than the regularly pruned ones.

> "A society grows great when old men plant trees whose shade they know they shall never enjoy" - Greek proverb

Masanobu drew the conclusion that pruning was only really necessary once the tree was already tampered with. I.e., once it was already accustomed to regular pruning, or if the tree had been grafted. He supposed that pruning should not be forsaken entirely, but to do so minimally, by removing any dead branches, and keeping the general shape of the tree the way nature intended.

I am wondering if the reason a tree puts out more fruit after heavy pruning each year, is because at some level it feels threatened. Subconsciously fearing for its life, it puts out fruit in order to continue its heritage. I've seen many cases where trees had stopped fruiting altogether, and a human has come along and decided to bulldoze them out. In two such cases the trees' root systems were stronger than anticipated, resulting in the farmer abandoning the quest. Leaving the trees half pushed over. The results were quite astounding. The following year, both trees fruited copiously! This is perhaps similar to when humans that have abused their bodies so much through bad diet, can't help themselves but spend much of their day obsessing about sex. Because deep down they are aware they are slowly killing themselves.

Richard StBarbe Baker

Another wonderful chap worth mentioning at this point, is "Richard StBarbe Baker". He understood far better than most the important role trees play, I mention him in passing as I was listening recently to an old radio broadcast from the late 1970s with him[138] (he was around 90 years old at the time. Well worth listening to!).

Manifesto

Planting fruit trees opens our hearts to nature's wisdom. Nurturing them gives exposure to life's vulnerabilities and teaches how to build ecological and human community.

> Planting fruit trees is about making love with the earth. Phantom planting works toward paradise. Let us live and love in paradise. Let us not be afraid to grow and change. Let us celebrate - life itself.

Fruit is the one food that is offered to us "free of charge". There is no taking of life, instead the fruit is offered as part of a symbiotic pact between plant, animal and the earth. The plant remains intact and benefits from the interaction. It gets to reproduce itself. What bliss, what joy! Not only does it get to reproduce through the sowing of its seed, but also the more delicious the fruit, the more chance we will nurture the seed, feed, water and care for it, until and after it brings to bare its own fruit.

Many people have never planted a fruit tree as they think they do not own land. But we are all children of the earth, we share equally in the valleys, hills rivers, seas. Let us no longer be deceived otherwise.

Phantom fruit tree planters have no formal organization, no joining fee. The earth alone holds its membership list throughout time. To belong, simply plant a fruit tree without expectation of material gain, help care for existing ones, or hold in your heart what they mean.

Is it too long to wait for an apple tree to grow? We do not need to live so fast that only instant results satisfy. Remember, we plant fruit trees not only for ourselves, but for those who will follow. Life gives unto life. By doing so, we can enjoy with clear conscience that which has been handed down from the past.

> "Until you dig a hole, you plant a tree, you water it and help it survive, you haven't done a thing. You are just talking." - Wangari Maathai

With due sensitivity, plant fruit trees on any land and in any place where they have a chance of surviving. We don't need permission. Nature sows without asking, and we are all part of nature. Reconstituting the world and working toward paradise is a duty and a right which extends beyond so called legal concepts of ownership.

Do not worry too much about losses. Accept these as part of the process. Take heart, knowing other fruit tree planters are also at work. What matters is not individual success or failure, but the overall process we share in.

TRANSITIONING

The Individual

When I think of transitioning, two seemingly contradictory Chinese proverbs spring immediately to mind. The first, *"great chasms cannot be jumped by two or more medium sized leaps"*, the second, *"even the journey of a thousand miles begins with a single step"*. It's irrefutably true, a great yawning chasm exists between shod omnivorism and Eden Fruitarianism and probably most people who are brave enough to attempt the jump fail, or spend years hanging on by their fingernails on the other side.

"Always remember that your present situation is not your final destination. The best is yet to come." - Unknown

I've seen people blogging on line, writing of their failed attempts and of their binges on pizzas, burgers and such. Now, although I think it's great they are so open and honest about their recurring lacks of success, I see it as pretty clear that they need to go back and rethink their strategy. I think it's an incredibly big ask for anyone to leap such a wide chasm, and it's likely that only the very, very rare, most ready, will ever succeed outright. For a raw food vegan of course the chasm has narrowed somewhat and such a leap has becomes much more feasible.

A healthy approach is to view Eden Fruitarianism not so much as a goal, but as a path whose ultimate destination is the utopia of Eden; a path bound predominantly by ethics and compassion, without which one can soon go astray.

"We cannot become what we want to be by remaining what we are." - Max DePree

By attempting to walk the path before one has even really succeeded at enlarging their circle of compassion to embrace animals is doomed to fail. One has to first really, and I mean *really*, really, realise that eating meat is comparable to paying someone to punch your next door neighbour in his face while you watch on and enjoy. In fact, I under-exaggerate, it's far worse! There are stun guns and knives and running blood and cold steel and prodding and cold jets of water and despair and faeces and urine and panic and foreboding and tortured moans and more suffering than you can shake a stick at. And that's just the last hours of an animals life. If you're stuck there and still feel diabolical urges to eat

204

zombilily, you need to educate yourself more, maybe visit a slaughterhouse. Maybe become vegan first but understand that there's a history behind that pizza that *you* are responsible for! Once the understanding has fully sunken in and taken root, it should be impossible to look at a burger in the same way. When you know there is no going back, re-evaluate fruitarianism, or consider a raw vegan diet. Find others at the same stage, on and off line, hook up with them so you can encourage each other and laugh and cry at your mistakes. Support is a good thing. Knowing you are not alone with your struggles can be of tremendous benefit to everyone. If you are genuinely committed to Eden Fruitarianism you will work on narrowing the chasmical gap and one fine day you will succeed in bridging it.

Many self christened fruitarians seem still to be unaware of their worldly ethical relationships. They still haven't done much with their circles of compassion, they are in it for health and fitness alone and their attitude is one of who really gives a damn if they might occasionally choose to eat a fish or a turkey. The fish does. The turkey[139] does. This is really the predominant reason I've coined this new term, Eden Fruitarianism; to make it clear that this is not about weight loss, healing or fitness. Although, to be sure, all three are much sought after by-products. Eden Fruitarianism is **NOT** a diet. It is above all, an awakening. It is not a goal, but a path toward ever increasing freedom, a path which cannot be followed without widening one's empathy and increasing one's understanding of ethics.

Addiction

A great deal of emotional investment is attached to cooked foods, and foods further

"I really regret eating healthy today." - No one.

down the priorly mentioned ethical food tower. Understanding emotional attachment is crucial to breaking free of it. Above all we should do our utmost to stay out of the bottom three layers, the flesh, the sentient life by-products and the grains. Although many may fall into the trap, try not to let yourself be fooled into viewing the likes of nuts, dried fruits, oils and superfoods as being valid Eden Fruitarian fare. Be aware of the instinctive stop. The subtle changes in the tastes and textures of food indicating it is time to push them aside. Once you have learned that commercial nuts, dried fruit, oils and superfoods are void of the *stop*, you will better understand why they should be avoided, which will thus better aid you in resisting their temptations.

The lower foods are often so devilishly addictive that we can easily mistake the hold they have over us as being the body crying out for proper sustenance. Remember it is rather like the cravings experienced by anyone coming off any heavy drug.

> Listening to your body, does not mean giving in to cravings!

Don't let lame and poorly thought through excuses deter you on your quest! If you find yourself irresistibly craving a food not eaten as offered by nature, then be sure the craving stems not from any genuine bodily need, but is surely more to do with addiction!

Understand that after defiling our internal temple, often beyond recognition of its one time splendour, there will, by necessity, be a period of detox. Many will likely also stumble at this stage and mistakenly believe detox to be a sign the Eden diet is not working for them. This is probably the biggest deterrent of all, stopping many in their tracks and making them announce to the world that they tried, but realised it just

> "No matter how many mistakes you make or how slow you progress, you are still way ahead of everyone who isn't trying." - Tony Robbins

wasn't for them. It's like their house is full of junk and waste and once they start to clean it out, all manner of cockroach, vermin and critters are disturbed from nesting amidst the piles of old pizzas cartons and discarded crusty underwear. You had no idea those critters were housing in there and once they start running around everywhere, you exasperatedly put up your hands and stop cleaning, Just look at the mess you've made. If you stop cleaning altogether, the vermin will settle back down again and things will return to a seemingly relative tranquillity. Yes, you are right, (I never fake a sarcasm), the dustpan and brush were a bad idea! Deep down, some will understand this, but nevertheless deny it and still see it as another good excuse to quit.

> If you are having trouble with "Will Power", try practising "Won't Power" Instead!

Coping With the Madness

As we awaken, the knowledge of the world being steeped in negativity becomes blatantly obvious. Wars, murder, corruption, self inflicted disease, poverty, injustice, mass slaughter of indisposed species bred purely for gluttonous purposes, babies left purposefully to cry "to teach them lessons" in goodness knows what, detrimental addictions and more. The list continues indefinitely with the madness inescapably surrounding us. It can be easy to become overwhelmed by it all, to become affected so deeply that we lose ourselves in the depravity of it all, lowering the quality of our own lives in the process. We may experience anger, frustration, hatred, pity and shame, or even feel so overburdened that we fall into fits of depression, and in so doing, we become lost.

Focusing on the negativity helps no one, least of all oneself. The key to success, and another great challenge for the Eden Fruitarian, is to be empathic without throwing one's own antagonistic thoughts into the equation. This will do nothing to ease or improve anything for anybody. There is no use in us being overwhelmed by empathy such that sadness rules our life. Somehow, we have to keep a positive attitude despite the negativity. To see the madness and move beyond it. To acknowledge its presence and do what we can to step out of it.

> "The mind has exactly the same power as the hands; not merely to grasp the world, but to change it." - Colin Wilson

The only consciousness we need to change is our own. By vanquishing mindful negativity, and our own destructive habits, we can encourage and pull others forward. If we can stay clear thinking and happy, despite the perplexities surrounding us, we set ourselves up as "examples" for the world to look up to. People will wonder "what's his/her secret?" and be inspired. If things get too heavy and at times they might, you need to step aside and focus on brighter things. See the treasures. Smell a flower, hug a good friend. go for a walk in the mountains. Close your eyes and relish the aromatic piquancy of a good durian. Lose yourself in the moment of bliss! Centre yourself in the now!

> Knowing what our goals are, is a matter of individual choice, keeping sight of them, is crucial to attaining them.

The Collective

What does this movement toward Eden mean in a broader community context? I've heard concern voiced more than once, over the quandary of "what if we all turned fruitarian tomorrow, how could the world cope?". Actually, when I first heard this question it was "what if we all turned *vegetarian* tomorrow, how could the world cope?". What would happen to all those cows and pigs and chickens and sheep? What would happen to all those dogs and cats if we suddenly forsook the pet industry altogether? People will argue that it is precisely because of these industries, that such animals have life in the first place, so surely this is a positive thing right?

207

Wrong! There is nothing "right" about any industry existing purely for profit, without genuine regard for the welfare of its sentient commodities. Do you think your life would be worth living if the entirety of it was spent incarcerated, if you were forcibly separated from your mother and family as a baby, fed poorly, had your movement restricted to the point where your muscles atrophied, where your life was ended prematurely after a long, hot, gruelling, packed ride with others all awaiting the same bloody destiny? There is no point or yearning desire for a predictable life void of freedom and any potential for inner growth. Don't try and kid yourself there is, and that you are somehow doing anyone a favour by having them experience this.

> "If it is important to you, you will find a way. If not, you'll find an excuse." - Unknown

It's likely that back when slavery was being challenged, there were supporters of the practice that would have argued the self same thing. You're putting slave owners out of business! Where would all the slaves go? What would they do without our support! No one can describe with any certain clarity how the world will look, while the reshuffle of order takes place. Big changes are needed and the fate of livestock animals must be effected. One thing is clear already, there is a gross overpopulation of farm animals, global statistics are not exactly easy to find, but it's estimated that the number of cattle alone is well north of a billion. In Australia there are just under 30 million (The number of people is less than 23 million!). I recall that the statistics from Norway, back when I lived there, were somewhat similar, with roughly one cow per inhabitant. Five million all up. No one really keeps tabs on chickens or how many of them there are world wide, but in Australia alone over 500,000,000 chickens are raised and slaughtered annually. The vast majority of them never even see the light of day! The approximate number of annually slaughtered pigs in Australia is five million. Anyone who continues to argue we are somehow doing any of these beings a favour by bringing them into existence and "letting them live" under the conditions they do, has clearly never really given this any considered ethical thought.

By stepping out of the picture and refusing to purchase consumer items necessitating bloody murder, you are not only washing your hands to it all, but helping toward cleaning up the planet from the mess we have made of it. Worrying about hypothetical "what ifs" serves no real purpose. If the whole of human society, the collective consciousness of mankind, should suddenly wake up and see the truth and have to deal with it, then I say: Let such a hypothetical world, deal with such an improbability. Trust that if it is hypothetically wise enough to experience a revelation of such magnitude, it would surely be wise enough to deal with its consequences too! We need also to be aware that the biggest issues will likely not so much be about a shortage in the production of fruit, but more to do with the distribution of the fruit. There is likely already more than enough fruit produced to feed the world, but greed and poor organisational skills prevent it from being distributed effectively. Globally, mountains of fresh produce are composted daily!

There is a passage in the bible[140] which states that toward the end, the world will suffer like a woman in labour, this will be inevitable, but once the time has passed, life will be so joyous, that all such suffering will soon fade in light of the bliss ahead. Okay, I may be taking liberties with the interpretation, but I call it how I see it and that's how it makes sense to me.

Conclusion

> The only evil that needs defeating, is the evil within ourselves.

Many will likely consider this chapter incomplete. I know the frustration of transition, the strong urges to fall back on old habits. Having passed through it all, I understand one might want further guidance of what to eat, when to eat and more, but the purpose of this book is to confirm our own self-reliance, and to show that such questions are for each of us alone to decide. This book identifies the path and offers inspiration. It is for you to seek further inspiration wherever and from whoever and whatever you can.

Ultimately the individual has to deal with their own issues. Misinformed choices have lead us to the situation we are in. Try to find others sharing your vision, connect with them however you can, and encourage each other. Hang in there! Grin and bare it! There is light at the end of the tunnel. Don't despair, be aware! If you genuinely feel a commitment to Eden Fruitarianism, you will find your way through the obstacles, I have every confidence success on this path is up for grabs for anyone who can truly understand the message I am sharing, and who truly desires to attain the goals they might set.

Truth, simplicity and love will be the team
that eventually ends all violence, bloodshed and wars.

TOPSY-TURVY WORLD

Life on Earth is currently inherently ailing, failing and flailing. This is something I believe we are all aware of to some extent. But because we are born into this sickness, a sickness so proliferous that it hides within itself, the true extent of such awareness is limited. Just how deep the ailing goes is mostly unrecognisable. Instead we come to consider the "ailing" as perfectly "normal" and that which differs greatly enough from that norm, to be both extreme and abnormal. This is what I call the Topsy-Turvy World. Where reality has moved so far from the truth, that the truth has become a lie and the lie a truth, leaving us all a confused, disturbed and basically troubled species, forever struggling with cognitive dissonance.

When I first became a vegetarian there was a general feeling amongst my then peers that I may have been a little over-sensitive and prone to exaggerating issues of morality. When I became vegan, I had gone totally over the top. I had become an extremist. On seeing the sense in raw and finally fruit, I most surely had lost all credibility with virtually everyone I knew. If I hadn't been of such otherwise sound mind, many would no doubt have wondered whether I was safe loose and caring for myself.

Of course, from my own perspective, with each new and blissful revelation, I was able to see with ever increasing clarity, just how intensely insane my original non thought through existence had been. From the stance of the shod omnivore, Eden Fruitarianism will undoubtedly be judged an extreme insanity by most. But from an Eden Fruitarian perspective, Shod Omnivorism is even more insane!

What was once considered normal and sane, has become abnormal and insane and that which once would have been considered insane, is now perfectly normally sane.

When we are accused of extremism, we can be quite sure it is often because the accuser has run out of better oppositional arguments. One may be considered extreme by

"What kind of messed up brainwashed society are we living in where exploitation and killing are considered 'normal' whereas compassion and non-violence are considered 'extreme'?"- Unknown

ceasing the intake of milk and eggs, despite the well-proven evidence of this being both a sound health choice, as well as an indisputably valid ethical one. Unable to logically counter these facts, opponents will thus often hide behind the torpid argument of "extremist".

The ideas expressed within this book are likely to be so distant from the reality perceived by most people, that they will find it difficult to agree with any of it.

I understand that. I face it every day. Which is why I try to centre myself with a non attached humour about it all. I wish there were a way for me to share my vision, such that people could understand that although distant from the reality of today, it is not without merit, and very worth striving for. I am a realist though, despite how you may think contrarily, and understand that unless one is ready, these words will fall into deaf ears, or blind eyes.

Sense of Smell

The things which we typically might think smell good, become foul smelling once one's body and mind

People go through life with the illusion that they really know shit. When in reality, they really know shit. Really, no shit! Just that tiny little syllabic stress of difference.

are cleansed enough. Naturally also (as is the very nature of Topsy-Turvyness), certain things that once smelt terrible will become more appealing than we ever thought possible. For an Eden Fruitarian to walk past a shop's decaying, cadaverous, meat and fish section, the odours are particularly, powerfully, unpleasantly pungent. Whereas the sweet fragrance of a durian is relished above many others. For many shod omnivores, the reverse is often quite true. Because the body is in a bad state of disrepair, all manner of sense inputs are confused and disorientated as a reflection of one's latent physiological unwellness.

Fresh bread, considered by probably most to be healthy and a basic daily necessity has an odour almost universally accepted as appealing. We are taught from a very young age how health beneficial bread is, especially wholemeal dark bread, and it's not at all easy to question that loyalty. However, once we do so, and have broken the addictive hold it has upon us, the attraction of the smell over time will gradually diminish until it becomes, as it rightly should, both unappealing and repulsive. Understanding the environmentally destructive nature of mono cereal crops should help to free us from any magical hold it may otherwise have on us.

As well as the confusing biblical "daily bread", there's the equally bizarre biblical prophecy of "the land of milk and honey". A symbol of rich fertile land for many, but taken literally, so very distant from a fruitarian Eden. The real rich fertility is to be found in the land of fruit and sunshine!

> "Many people consider a raw food diet to be radical. Yet there are roughly 1,800,000 species that eat raw food, and only one that eats cooked." - Unknown

Treats

In order to incite our children to behave well, we often use the psychology of "treats". Stop crying and you can have some cake. Be a good boy and you can have an ice-cream. "I've worked so hard, I deserve a bar of chocolate and a nice chilled glass of champagne to swill it down". "I've been so good eating raw all week, I deserve some roast potatoes". If only the truth were unveiled and the bigger picture more visible. We are brainwashed into thinking of such foods as something good, something we earn, something positive. So far from the addictive health detrimental reality of the unbiased truth.

> "If fifty million people say a foolish thing, it is still a foolish thing." - Bertrand Russell

False labelling

We have this big thing about "organic food" where it is clearly labelled as such. This surely shows the extent of our fall. Surely it should be organic food which is "normal", and all the other foods should be labelled and marked with whatever chemicals and poisons that were diabolically added and used during their production?

Narrow-mindedness?

The extent of the madness goes far beyond what we eat though, it goes far beyond being told we are inflexible and narrow-minded, when we as Eden Fruitarians, know the reverse is really true and that we would never have reached Eden Fruitarianism had we been anything remotely resembling inflexible or narrow minded! It goes with all aspects of society that we initially regard as normal, purely because "that's the way it is".

Make-up and body paints

Take make-up as an example. Somehow we have been sold the lie it makes us look more attractive. This idea is so ingrained into the mass consciousness of humanity, that regular daily application is considered by many to be perfectly normal. People absorbing goodness knows what toxicity through their lips and facial skin, and looking only messed up and scummy from the process. Such is the perspective of the Eden Fruitarian. Suddenly you recognise the king is in fact naked!

Now, if someone massaged papaya skin into their face, or mango skin over their body, there would be stifled embarrassed laughter, from those who will see such an insanity as a profanity. In such cases though, one would not even leave it on all day, but follow shortly with a quick dip in fresh flowing water!. Once more, the normal is abnormal and the abnormal, normal.

Nudism

Nudism, and the art of soaking up sunlight is conventionally viewed as slightly eccentric at best, to downright permissive and degenerate at worst. However, the nudist considers it a liberating and health giving pastime, and behaviour to be expected on hot summer days. We also see the perversion inherent in the often shared mass psyche that open nudity somehow automatically equates to public sex.

The real Mafia

Then there's hair and shoes and appearances and laws, don't get me started on laws, created by the world's greatest criminal organisations. So cleverly have they infiltrated our existence, that we've been lead to believe that we can't thrive without them. I am of course talking of the governments and politicians, the most corrupt venture on the planet. Making criminals and prisoners of those who oppose. Banning us from walking freely by enforcing artificial borders. The opposite to such a

213

state of affairs is seen as "lawlessness" and anarchy, often falsely thought to equate to widespread uncontrolled violence and pillage. Sadly, the shod omnivores might be on to something there, we have collectively created an environment where the absence of big brother just seems far too challenging for most.

A shepherd is needed to guide his sheeple flock. Yet another topsy-turvy point, as most think of the shepherd as playing a kind beneficial role, the protector, the guider, the provider. And although he may be all those things, it is only to an extent and not without ulterior motive. Cut to the chase, and the one true reason the

> "The greatest enemy of knowledge is not ignorance, it is the illusion of knowledge" - Stephen Hawking

shepherd cares for his flock, is exploitative. He does not keep the wolf at bay so you can live a long, prosperous and happy life of liberty. He does so, in order that he alone may reap the benefits of the sheeple flesh and hides. The shepherd guiding his flock is such a poor cliché!

No, the Eden Fruitarian sees beyond the need to be governed and strives to live in a truly unfettered realm. Many will rule him unrealistic and having his head in the clouds, but he acknowledges once more the topsy-turvy nature of such realism. Much as the imminence of global change (for the better) may indeed be slim, continuing to dream the way the masses do, will only serve to push us closer toward the brink of annihilation. By adopting Eden Fruitarianism, one is effectively moving on, and looking positively toward a brighter more peaceful future, where the only valid laws are spiritual ones; the need to treat all life with the respect it deserves, and that we ourselves may rightly also expect.

> FAST - not Feast.
> FRUIT - not Flesh.
> FIG - not Fish.
> FRESH - not Fowl.

But back to the government, who insist it is illegal to print your own money, to create your own passport, to sell drugs, to bear arms, to imprison and to kill. That is of course if you are not part of, or affiliated with, that organisation. It matters not what other names they may go by, the Illuminati[141], the Bilderbergers[142], the trilateral commission[143], or the knights of the scimitar[f], the crux of the matter is they are a self appointed legalised Mafia crime syndicate that have made it seem like resistance is futile and that we are powerless to oppose them.

---

f   This one's a reference to an episode from the sit-com "Cheers".

214

Peddling drugs and Vaccination

Peddling drugs is an illegal activity and yet through their so called "health institutions", they are peddled daily. And then there is alcohol, considered by most to be a perfectly acceptable and normal addition to one's social life. On the other hand, those who sell and use marijuana are considered criminals and punished, sometimes quite severely so, for their belligerent behaviour. And yet, although deaths related to alcohol intake are comparatively common[144], similar deaths related to marijuana are virtually unheard of! Marijuana is said to be illegal because it is supposedly dangerous and health threatening, but the real reason is it cannot so easily be controlled by the mega-corporations. If it were purely a question of health risks, the consumption of both tobacco and alcohol would also be prohibited.

> The Pioneer mind achieves its object in the end by educating and by reaching the latent altruism of others, until what began as the insight of the exceptional few, becomes the shared vision of an awakened social conscience.

Don't get me wrong, I'm not by any means trying to condone marijuana nor any other mind altering drug, I am merely showing the insanity inherent within the collective consciousness of society. The persuasion that leads to acts of legalisation, to make easily available and push one of the most toxic drugs[145] onto the masses, while users of comparatively less harmful ones are victimised.

> "If you are always trying to be normal, you will never know how amazing you can be!" - Maya Angelou

While still on the subject of drugs, yet another example of topsy-turvyness springs to mind, once more stemming from the practices of the Mafia (that is, the government) supported drug peddlers. Vaccines[146]. The shod omnivorous masses tend to just accept what they are told and unquestioningly herd their children to be jabbed. With unwavering faith many will themselves queue up to receive their annual flu injections. All it takes though, is a little research[147] to reveal the darker side and reveal that things aren't quite as the powers that be, would have us seem. Delve deeper, and you'll find vaccinations to be not even vegan friendly, with all manner of animal abuse behind their development and constitution. Here in Australia, the 2013 elections are advertising a financial penalty for those who refuse to conform!

If you have full confidence in vaccines[148], and plan on getting vaccinated, or vaccinating your own children, at least download and print this PDF file first[149]. I am told that physicians will refuse to sign it. I wonder why?

Sunlight

And sunlight, now there's something. We are taught in a way to fear it. To seek out the shade instead of the light, to go over to the dark side! As a result, reports are now coming in that health is being jeopardise through low vitamin D[150]. That's a good thing though right? It means the sale of Vitamin D pills will increase!

TV and Media

Taking media and TV as a final example. We have become so conditioned to thinking and accepting violence as normal, that virtually everything we read and see is based around it. From the nature programs that are mostly about how animals hunt, or are hunted, how they band together in flocks for safety and in packs to terrorise, how the wildebeest play Russian roulette crossing the crocodile infested river and how the hyenas single out the weak of the herd before ripping it to shreds. Many get their kicks out of such shows of ferocity and aggression. Fiction TV usually includes someone getting killed at some point, often it's the focal point of the whole story line!

Weird is the new normal.

The Aquarius Pandemic

Recently, as I lay down to sleep, I had a sudden flash of inspiration. An idea for a movie, or a possibly hit TV series. The next morning I woke up and hurriedly wrote down the basic outline synopsis. I christened the story, "The Aquarius Pandemic":

It begins with a young Aussie surfer. A happy chappy with few real concerns or issues in his life. Let's call him "Sunny". He lives in Victoria on the south coast.

He has a gift. A gift he has, up until now, been completely unaware of. It is the gift to recognise enlightenment.

Sunny's life changes when one evening he goes to attend a talk given by a woman named Mara. Mara is an enlightened being and the first Sunny has ever encountered. She talks of empathy, of letting go of fear, and of the need for us to stop using peer pressure as excuses for what we do. For us to end the sheeple mentality and to begin taking responsibility for our actions, be more aware. He is shaken by the talk and sees her enlightenment as a burning flame, something he has never before seen in anyone and becomes fascinated by that flame.

After returning home, he blogs about his encounter. It is not long before others begin to comment on his blog and write of other supposedly enlightened beings scattered around the globe.

Driven by his urge to be once more in the presence of "the flame", he sets out on a backpacking/surfing holiday, and a quest to find and meet others, whose flames are alight.

> "It's better to walk alone, than in a crowd going in the wrong direction!"
> - Diane Grant

Over a five year period, he travels to over twenty different countries, meeting over thirty people, all of whom make some claim to enlightenment. Blogging his experiences and insight as he goes. Through his unique gift, he immediately recognises many of them as charlatans. Nevertheless he discovers that eight of them genuinely have the flame.

He returns broke to Victoria after his trekking and has a plan; to reunite the eight awakened gurus.

Cutting a long story short, an anonymous donor (through the blog), pays for the eight to come together.

This is the first time in human history for enlightened people to actually meet one another. For Sunny, the effect of so many flames at once serves to ignite his own inner flame, and he now becomes the world's ninth enlightened being.

> "People are fed by the food industry, which pays no attention to health, and are treated by the health industry which pays no attention to food." - Wendell Berry

The reason Sunny was able to recognise the flame of enlightenment was largely due to the fact that he himself was on the verge of enlightenment. Only fellow enlightened beings have the ability to truly recognise the flame of another's enlightenment. Which of course, as explained, was a hitherto unknown occurrence, as no two enlightened gurus had until then ever met, or been in the presence of another.

The nine sit down together and a joint decision is made to concentrate their efforts in awakening the rest of the world.

DAY 1 - POPULATION OF EARTH 8 billion and counting (show ever increasing number).

Number of enlightened beings - Nine.

Show the planet. Hone in on an army base outside of Fortworth, Texas. A sergeant is barking orders at a bunch of stiffly standing soldiers (standing next to their beds in a dorm). Suddenly his voice is faded out in the mind of one soldier. You can see a look of realisation growing on him and he eases out of his stiff stance and looks around at his fellow troopies. The Sergeant notices this sudden change in stance and attitude and walks over to the lad barking loudly. The soldier stays relaxed and answers calmly. He no longer needs anyone to tell him what to do and how to stand. Even after the sergeant gets more physical, the lad manages to stay calm throughout and talking rationally insisting that he think and do for himself. Of course, this ends up with the soldier having his arse dragged out of there, but all along at an unthinkable peace with his treatment.

> "People say you are mad, do you know that? When you went off to war they said you were fine, intelligent - and now you are mad, because... because you sing like the birds, you chase after butterflies and... you look at flowers. I think you were mad before, not now."
> Claire - Brother Sun, Sister Moon

Show the planet again. Hone in on some random place in Iran. A halal butcher, busy chopping up the carcass of a dead lamb. Blood on his apron, stress on his face. Suddenly his demeanour changes, he puts down his hacker and begins thinking. He sees the life of the lamb and the terror of her final moments, and no longer wants to be a part of it. He walks away from it all.

> "All your duties are included in this: Do nothing to others that would pain you if it were done to you" - Mahabharata

Show the planet again. Hone in on some random city in Europe. A house. A woman. She is getting dressed. Opens her shoe cupboard, stares at her shoes, selecting a pair to match her outfit. Suddenly she awakens and sees her large selection of shoes as humorously insane. She smiles. Looks at herself in the mirror, shakes her head, touches the lipstick and make-up on her face in wonderment. She washes it off.

Another planet shot. Another random country. A man leaving to work, dressed in his fancy suit. He gets onto the street in his car, drives shortly, before awakening. Pulls over with that realising look on his face. Turns around and returns home. His wife is shocked to hear he has decided to quit work, that he sees no value in what he does. Have them talking something other than English, with subtitles. I want to make it clear, what is happening is global.

Planet again. Pick a country. This time a border guard official who is preventing someone from entering the country. After awakening, she realises she has no right to stop someone moving wherever they wish. Despite not having all their ducks in a row, she lets the person pass.

> "The difficulty is to free the mind from the known so that it can discover what is new all the time" - J. Krishnamurti

Basically this can continue and shows people all over the planet awakening and realising how their lives have been pointless or exploitive. These people all become rational and calm and share the fact they no longer fear authority. They no longer need to take orders, or have someone else think for them. They know the true value of life, a value they have hitherto neglected. They no longer wish for their lives to be a burden on others, or cause unnecessary suffering to others, this includes animals too and from henceforth they question everything they eat and do. They see things more vividly for what they really are.

Have the people be of both genders and random age and ethnicity. Even children.

DAY 2 - Population of the world -show the ticker counter thing,

Number of Enlightened humans - 16

> "It is forbidden to kill; therefore all murderers are punished, unless they kill in large numbers and to the sound of trumpets" - Voltaire

So, day one basically sparked another seven awakenings around the globe. Day two can continue likewise. A hunter taking aim at a deer, suddenly sees what he is doing and looks at the rifle he carries seeing it as a tool of destruction. He buries it. A rich man being driven by his chauffeur realises their equality and asks the driver to stop so that he may move to the front of the limo and talk with the servant as an equal. A priest at mass suddenly realising what religion is, changes his sermon to talk of how all religions have it wrong and that the real spirituality comes from within and self awareness and of questioning everything.

A homeless bag man pushing his shopping cart full of plastic bags of rubbish he is clinging too, he lets go. An obese woman, eating suddenly looks at her plate and sees her reflection (she is not angry with herself, or ashamed, just slightly bewildered as to how she got there, but can see clearly how to move on). A doctor is sitting with a patient about to vaccinate a child, on awakening he tells the truth and states honestly, there is no way he would vaccinate his own child.

Similar occurrences around the globe. Have people awakening and seeing not only the follies of their own existence, but also how the planet has been ravaged and savaged through the pursuit of material gain with no thoughts to spirituality or environmental consequences. It needs to be shown, the pounding the planet has taken during the last 200 years since world domination has been the goal of the global elite. How much forest has been devastated and how other species have suffered. The awakened ones can see it all. It is all clear to them. But they are not wallowing in pity or shame or negativity. They are just able to see and stop being a part of it.

With the number of enlightened people almost doubling daily, with some joining the original nine. After one week the government(s) and military have begun to recognise this international happening and have christened it "the Aquarius pandemic". They are not happy.

There are also some who have begun to take advantage of the situation. They see the people that are awake as easy pushovers, only passively resisting, thus when their material possessions are removed from them, they don't physically protest, just offer words of wisdom spoken calmly. Pearls before swine.

> "The quieter you become, the more you can hear. Silence is not the absence of something, but the presence of everything." - Gordon Hempton

The government is desperate to stop whatever it is that is happening and the original awakened soldier is under lock and key being questioned and prodded.

The identity of the original nine is discovered, and the location invaded. The roughly thirty people they find there, are all separated and taken captive, but by this time it is far too late, many other groups of enlightened people have joined together around the globe and begun to collectively focus their creative thoughts and energies toward healing the planet through awakening others.

There can be a lot going on with government people doing their darnedest to put a stop to it, but resistance is ultimately futile as they also, slowly awaken.

As the numbers of awakened people increase exponentially, with finally more gurus than sheeple, it is self evident, the city is not the place to be. The whole system as we currently know it has collapsed. People are NOT reaching for their guns as is the traditional case in similar scenarios, they are seeing their guns as inherently destructive and burying them. They are NOT banding together creating territorial outlaw communities and greedily raiding stores for supplies and equipment. As the planet finally is all engulfed by the flames of enlightenment, there is no more fear. No more need to be controlled and governed. All corruption is a thing of the past. Communities arise and focus is on gardening and planting fruit trees. Re-Edenising the planet.

> Doctor: "Don't forget, you are what you eat."
> Patient: "In that case I need to eat a skinny person."

Long suppressed clean technologies are finally released and replace all destructive technology. Despite enlightenment, people still have talents they wish to exercise, but instead of using money as a means to get what they want, people basically just do as they wish and IT WORKS!

Okay, there can be a couple of underlying stories throughout the chronicle, following maybe Sunny and the soldier and maybe the first guy who returned home and told his wife that he was no longer working, but basically this is it. What do you reckon, does it have potential? Maybe the anonymous donor could be a rich visionary we witness following the blog of Sunny. Focus on Sunny's own coming of awareness too.

Know any film producers? Someone influential enough in TV and who might be willing to consider the idea? Please feel free to share around. The world has fully embraced the dark side and desperately needs to step into the light.

Never give up on a dream, just because its manifestation will take time. Time does not stop.

COMPROMISES

The mind realisation of Eden Fruitarianism is a momentous one, but after the dust of the moment has settled and the task of following its path looms dauntingly ahead, it is easy to lose oneself in the difficulty and immensity of the undertaking involved. Virtually every aspect of human existence, indeed existence in general, is currently, at least partially, exploitative and contrary to a vision of Eden. This may make the path seem futile, but this would just be lazy thinking inspired from the dark side. We need to move into the light regardless of how dull it is and how often it wavers and understand the more we seek it, the stronger its luminosity, and the less it will flicker, making the path ever clearer.

> "A dead fish can float downstream, but it takes a live one to move against the current!"- W.C. Fields

Meanwhile though, there will be unavoidable compromises one must make. To begin with, it is quite likely that one finds oneself in a "normal" job, in an urban setting, often with a daily commute to and from work involved. One's choice of food may appear at first to be poor and a hindrance toward pursuing one's dream, or addiction so strong and peer/family pressure so powerfully influential that positive changes will struggle arduously against the grain of everything and everyone around you. Like you are swimming upstream and not getting anywhere.

There are two main aspects which need to be understood with compromises. The first is to not let them deter you and the second is to not use them as excuses to compromise yet further. The more you make an effort, the easier it will be to find valid solutions.

Short of abandoning civilisation entirely and moving completely off the grid, some compromises may forever be unavoidable, purely because there is no clean valid alternative. Besides, realistically, moving fully off the grid, will likely also entail initial compromises, as "off the grid" there is currently very little for a budding Eden Fruitarian to eat.

> "Could you look an animal in the eyes and say to it: 'My appetite is more important than your suffering'?" - Moby

Not relying on fossil fuel driven vehicles for example, is a practical improbability. Of course, we can lighten our carbon footprint by getting around as much as practically possible with a push-bike and a sturdy set of back panniers, but we're still reliant on our food being delivered to the shops and stalls we purchase from and the further we are from the source of our food, the less we are likely to know of its history and origins.

If there genuinely isn't enough choice of fruit available though, make sure you still eat as high on the food tower as you are able, and look for ways to forever improve those choices. This will naturally involve effort on your behalf, you'll have to make your desires known to the world around you, perhaps start by growing your own tomatoes in a window box, or even consider relocating as an option, we have to be the change we wish to see in the world!

When you are ready, committed and enthused enough, it is best to move to an area where there is more choice, or better yet, to an area where that choice is grown locally, or to where you have land to grow at least some of your own food.

Even after you have been on the path for a while, there will likely always be compromises of some form on another.

Adopt a fruit diet and help humanity and all life, evolve toward the light side!

In our own personal circumstances, although we grow some of our own food, we are still a way off from being self sufficient and live in remote enough an area (to escape the yahooing of shod zombie omnivores and the urban madness of barking dogs and incessant lawn-mowing), that we currently can't practically manage without using a car for supplies and such.

We know it's not ideal, but we don't despair about it. We do the best we can and aim toward ever lessening the necessity of fuel consumption. If this world could straighten itself out and more people grew more fruit around us, the need for a vehicle or questionable food suppliers, could be diminished yet further. We all need to work together on this.

"We have all come from the One Great Spirit, and this precious earth is our common mother. Let us walk in Harmony.." - Native Wisdom

As an aside, even this book is in some ways a compromise of my morals. I'm stuck behind a computer screen aware I am doing injury to my arms and eyes and posture in the process. I am debating with myself whether or not I should have it published on paper and although I know once more it isn't ideal, am strongly considering doing so. I feel the message is sufficiently important enough to merit the paper, even though part of me struggles with the regret I will feel in doing so.

It is true, we still buy some fruit from supermarkets, thus some of it not as locally sourced as would be preferred. This world makes it difficult to follow one's ideals to the T. But the important thing with compromises is to be aware of them, and to move forward with one's spirit to be one day rid of them. Remember Eden Fruitarianism is a path, not a goal. The goal is Eden.

> "Be kind whenever possible. It is always possible."- Dalai Lama

With the current state of worldly affairs, there is generally uncertainty of whether one's food is grown, picked and distributed correctly, unless of course one grows it oneself. There are the issues with a whole host of chemicals used as fertilisers, pesticides, herbicides etc. Even the certified organic food has its issues, the blood and bone and similar (by)products from the animal abuse industry. The destructive mono crop methods most frequently employed, the borderline slave labour task force, working to harvest and prune etc, the inefficient methods of distribution and much more. There's even the issue of dishonesty concerning the history of food. There are foods sold as organic which are not, and foods sold as local which are not.

Even if we have land, and passion to grow our own foods, the highly tuned empathy of the Eden Fruitarian will soon realise there are compromises there too. For those who took the time to watch the Myth Buster's Video I mentioned earlier in the book[151], or those who are already sensitive enough to be aware of plant perception, once one sits down and works mindfully on a garden, one becomes aware of actions and their effects. There is an inevitable need to weed out grasses and other plants growing in the wrong places. Short of becoming breatharian, there is no current way around this dilemma. However, through "growing it oneself" one can be infinitely more aware of all steps involved. Weeding can be minimised by using newspaper layering, and mulching and communicating with the plants as one does so. They WILL hear you!

> "The only man who never makes a mistake, is the man who never does anything."
> - Theodore Roosevelt

It is our task to inform ourselves, as best we are able and to make the best choices we can based on that information. Until the world sorts itself out, the best choice is to grow whatever we can ourselves and to *not let compromises deter us on our path*!

224

BENEFITS OF EDEN FRUITARIANISM

1. You'll have a clean conscience with all animal exploitation, including the bred victims of the pet trade.
2. You'll be doing your part to help restore the environment.
3. Your food choice is the least harmful of all.
4. No cooking involved. Thus no need for pots and pans etc.
5. No oils involved.
6. You'll stop the harming of your body caused by eating inferior foods.
7. You'll be helping rid yourself of karmic debt.

> "Those who were seen dancing were thought to be insane by those who could not hear the music." - Nietzsche

8. You'll save time with food preparation and clean up.
9. You'll save electricity due to the no cooking.
10. You'll find yourself generating a lot less rubbish, even the potential to completely cut it out.
11. Fruit cleanses as well as nourishes us and will eventually bring us all to our ideal weight.
12. Fruit helps keep our body supple.
13. Fruit gives us a mental clarity and nurtures a spiritual well being.
14. Fruit reduces the amount of water needed and keeps us well hydrated.
15. Unlike many of the other foods, ripe fresh fruit is completely none addictive and always accompanied by the instinctive stop.
16. Fruit is the best tasting of all raw foods.
17. Fruit is the most colourful and pleasing to the senses.
18. Bowel movements will be predictably regular.
19. The toilet waste of a fruitarian is far less offensive and, without treatment, is a welcome addition to the soil in one's garden. (you'll have tomatoes popping up everywhere!).
20. You'll find yourself sleeping better, with dreams being less chaotic.

> "Believe you can, and you're halfway there." - Theodore Roosevelt

21. Being barefoot, you'll be more connected with the earth.
22. And receiving permanent foot zone therapy!
23. Your energy levels will increase.

24. You won't need all those cleansing products, or can at least avoid them as much as possible.
25. An empty bathroom cabinet.
26. Suddenly 90 - 95% of the supermarket will become irrelevant.
27. Virtually no regular need for doctor or dentist intervention.
28. No more annual/biannual colds. (The germs have no lasting interest in a clean body!).
29. No need for barbers and hairdressers. Perfumes, deodorants and make up.
30. If practised properly and from an early enough age, it should ensure a long and happy life.
31. All pain will be lessened.
32. Flowers will smell nicer.
33. You will smell nicer.

MISCELLANEOUS MUSINGS

You might be mistaken in thinking that were I to rule the world, I would abolish many things, but such thoughts are far from my mind. I would not ban slaughterhouses, nor carnivorous animals, nor drugs, nor force the world to be vegan. Prohibition just sends industries underground, making them seedier and darker.

> Why should politicians be buried at least ten meters underground? - Because deep down, they are really good people.

However, were I to be able to guide the world, while it is still in the clutches of darker forces, I would encourage ethics as a compulsory school subject and support the global need for gaining and nurturing much needed empathy. Through media and maybe financial incentive for script writers to write enthralling stories, focusing less on guns and punches, and more on the light side.

> Homer: Don't blame me, *I* voted for Kodos.

Politics

Politically, while government structures still exist, I'd like to see some kind of enforced accountability for promises made that are not kept. Especially when voiced intentions turn out clearly to have been nothing more than mendacious vows. The simple commandment of *thou shalt not lie,* should be honoured by all those in positions of popular trust, and those who disobey this law, should be publicly humiliated at best. This needs to be rigidly enforced, and those it concerns need to be closely monitored at all times. Perhaps it would make some think twice before entering an occupation, where one can so easily be corrupted. I am not entirely ignorant of the enormity of such an undertaking; who will police the police? I believe with enough forethought, there is a possibility of such a proposition becoming reality and functioning efficiently.

> Interesting anagram of "Election Results" - Lies, let's recount

What I'd also like to see change with the political system, is its method of election. Of course, the ultimate goal is to be rid of such systems altogether, but while they are still around, changes are crucial to moving forward. Instead of this "one man, one vote" system, which most of us with half a brain or more can see is a bit of a farce, I propose a "one man, multiple vote" election system. Let's take a scenario, let's suppose, there are the following seven contenders, Conservative, Labour, Liberal, the Greens, the Socialists, the National Front and the Loonies. Instead of just choosing one of them, as would be the normal "democratic" scenario, Let's say I can now give each party a point between +5 and -5 and that only one can get each number. I am convinced in such an electoral system, provided the results remain unfudged, the results would offer a much more honest representation of what the populace truly wants. A truly proportional representation! Naturally, only parties that receive an overall positive set of points can represent.

When I suggested this to a friend some years ago, explaining initially that a new system could be something more similar to the way the Eurovision song contest winners are elected, she guffawed and answered "But there's a completely unpredictable new winner every year!". Yes, because they sing different songs every year! This should not be the case with political parties.

Also, I believe it would be quite fair to make the wages of politicians hover around the countries mean wage. I guess I really mean 'median wage', not the really mean minimum one! This would surely give them incentive to raise the median, and weed out those who are purely after money and power!

> I never wanted to believe that my dad was stealing from his job as a road worker. But when I got home, all the signs were there.

Family

We have a chauvinistic family name system, which is pretty much always centred around the male of the family. Mr. Rolland marries Ms Northcutt, who henceforth becomes Mrs Rolland and any children they may conceive take on the father's name too. Some of the more liberated women might keep their name, or in rare instances, the husband may adopt the name of the wife instead, however, much as on the surface it may seem the woman's name is taken, all they have done is taken on the male name from the mother's side, the father of the bride's name. This has been going on for as far as the history books show. My proposition is we suspend with this clearly male dominant practice and instead do something creative and fun. Let's say, when a couple marry, they are given free range to come up with a new name that is a partial anagram of their two family names combined. Thus in the above scenario, they will not become Mr & Mrs Rolland, but combining Rolland and Northcutt together, become something like Mr & Mrs Latchron. They should give it as much combined thought as they would do to naming their children.

As is the case with most of my ever-so brilliant ideas, when I've tentatively suggested this in the past, people have laughed and said it would make tracing one's family tree back a nightmare. I counter with two, I believe very valid, points; 1. In this current digitally obsessed era, it should be no problem to keep clear tabs on whose called what, and when they changed their names etc. And more importantly, 2. Tracing one's family tree is really a bit of a joke anyway, especially along the father's father's (etc.) line, as the chances of infidelity increase exponentially for each generation. Go back ten generations and you can be pretty darned sure that that guy was not really your great great, great etc. grand father at all, regardless of what any paperwork says, the chances are incredibly slim. The further you go back, the slimmer the chances, so although there may be a theoretical likelihood that Louis the fourteenth has descendants alive today, anyone that has traced their family back and found him to be their ancestor is, with all probability and likelihood, misinformed.

While you ponder over the significance of that, I'm going to jump to another branch of controversy.

Breatharianism

When I first began outlining this book, I had tentatively arranged to have a Breatharianism chapter following the

> After smelling the cherry blossoms, I sighed - *Beautiful!* And a spray of tiny petals went twirling in my breath.
> - Allan Hart

Eden Fruitarianism one. After giving it more thought, I decided against doing so. Although I've undergone several fasts of varying lengths, I have always done so with the intent of resuming eating later, and thus never seriously attempted to live purely on air. I've been fascinated by the idea of breatharianism for the past couple of decades though, and although I have yet to personally meet anyone who I can confirm genuinely does not eat, I nevertheless still believe such a state of being is indeed possible.

However, despite this lacking of first hand experience, I still feel like throwing in my tuppence worth, hence I've made room for it here, in this subsection, together with a hodgepodge of other mismatched notions. Perhaps later when I feel more certain or confident in my own viewpoint on this, I will revise this section and separate it into its own deserved chapter. Or delete it altogether.

Before you get over emotional and heated about how ridiculous the concept of living on love, light and fresh air might appear to you, please take time out to consider the following:

Firstly, there are unquestionably some out there who claim to be living on air and water alone[152]. (And undoubtedly Love, Light and Hugs too). As said, I cannot personally vouch for the authenticity of any of these claims, but nevertheless I strongly suspect there are a good number trying, and some truth to at least a percentage of those claims.

> Nappies and politicians should be changed often. Both for the same reason.

Secondly, if any mature person should decided to follow a path of breatharianism, then it is fully their own choosing. I see three possible outcomes to such a choice. 1, They may not succeed, but may die in the process. 2, They may not succeed and return to more solid substances once more. and 3, They may succeed and move on to something higher. In any of the three scenarios, only the individual is at risk.

Thirdly, a far more grisly, greasy fact, is that those at the complete other extreme, the shod omnivores who eat the flesh of others daily, do not only put themselves at risk. Indeed, given let's say, a below average lifespan of sixty years, it is quite (un)reasonable that a human flesh-eater might in that span of time, devour the equivalent of something like six hundred chicken carcasses, fifteen cows, forty pigs, forty sheep, possibly thousands of fish and countless other animals. I'm likely underguestimating, one website offers the ballpark figure of sixteen thousand animals consumed over the average lifetime of an American meat eater[24]. To be sure, the average zombie dawn of the living dead flesh-eater puts the butchered burnt remains of hundreds of thousands of animals into their stomach. What a graveyard! - R.I.P!

> Eat sunlight, live long and prosper.

Think of all the misery and suffering this "choice" causes! This is only the fleshy side of things; include dairy and eggs and who knows the true extent of deaths and suffering of individuals the average westernised human might be causing!

How many people have died from alcohol related incidents, and in hospital beds daily, from cancers, heart diseases and old-timers. All predominantly diet related.

So how could such a hypothetical state of being a breatharian, ever be attained you might ask? Well, there are several theories I have come across that may shed some light. To begin with, biological transmutation seemed the most likely to me [see the section by that name in the Eden Fruitarianism chapter]. Recently though, I have been corresponding with a guy claiming to be breatharian in South America. His theory is that a fully cleansed body ultimately needs no material sustenance. He is not the first to propose this, as Hilton Hotema[153] frequently made mention of much the same in his books, particularly "Man's Higher Consciousness"[154]. It makes for fascinating reading.

Then there is the practice of "sun gazing"[155], which many claim if practised long and regularly enough can eventually lead not only to increased energy levels, but also to the body no longer requiring food of any kind. Although it is easy to immediately dismiss the idea, as it sounds rather far fetched and the risk of eye damage quite serious, there are all the same a growing number of people practising the technique claiming to receive varied benefits[156] least of which being the lessening for requirement of physical nourishment.

> "When I let go of what I am, I become what I might be" - Lao Tzu

Personally, I do not recommend anyone to try breatharianism without first being of fully sound mind and body. Doing so otherwise will likely result in failure. Failure may be a likely result regardless of this, but if you are of sound mind, you can at least cease the experiment should it be clear it is failing. In every case, I would never recommend anyone to attempt breatharianism unless they have moved to the top floor of the ethical food tower and have proven to themselves, they are able to live healthily and happily, for at least a few years, on solely fruit. No exceptions. That is, in order to step onto the roof of the food tower, to fully transcend food, fruit is likely the gateway.

Why would anyone wish to transcend solid sustenance entirely, when most people would probably look at the idea as being a painful deprivation? The thought of not eating all those 'good' things one has become accustomed (addicted) to is probably not a pleasant one. Food has become such an issue in all our lives, we are probably all guilty of overeating, so quite profoundly, how can we even expect to live without eating, when we can't even live without overeating?

For me, the breatharian path is about letting go. It's about understanding we are more than just gross physical manifestations. It's about accepting our true potential and once we learn to transcend the newly proposed tower, all that is left is air, love, light and material independence. Presumably this would give us the freedom to explore, to walk unfettered in any direction. To boldly go, where no one has gone before. Well, perhaps nearly no one.

Military

I believe this idea was first suggested by Peace Pilgrim[157], but worth including here as it's still

> A soldier who's been through mustard gas and pepper spray, is a seasoned veteran.

as valid. She suggested that instead of the military focusing on devastation and serial killing, the army could be responsible for monitoring and cleaning land pollution, the navy could do likewise with the water ways[158] and the air-force could clean up the air ways pollution. What a great idea!

Prisons and Schools

Both are symptoms of a sick society. I don't believe in oppressing symptoms and wouldn't dream of doing so with these ones either, but it's worth acknowledging, neither would be around in a more healthy world. Crime is pretty much inevitable once you group so many people together that we no longer even know who our next door neighbours are. If cities and large towns broke up and we all moved into smaller more tightly knit communities with more emphasis put on growing our own food, (especially fruit trees), and meaningful social interaction and ethics, then crime would inevitably diminish.

> "To learn who rules over you, simply find out who you are not allowed to criticise." - Voltaire

For me, school was an ordeal, often a nightmare, I perceived we were all being trained to be good little society slaves, or army drones, even the uniforms drove this home. Learning was a struggle, as much of what was forced upon us, was really not very interesting. Or presented in ways that watered our boredoms. This was not just an issue of having terrible teachers in oversized classrooms, the whole school system seemed wrong to me.

I'm not proposing children not be taught anything, but in smaller more manageable sized communities, I believe teaching would be an every day aspect of living and all adult members would be a part of that process, teaching kids the basic necessities of life and whatever else they naturally have a flare for. Especially I believe the most important subject of all should be on empathy and ethics. Teach children to recognise other sentient life forms, including plant perception. Show them nature's art, expressed through flowers and how the plant objects if we rob it of its expressiveness by forcibly separating the flower from the plant.

In any case, while schools exist in the general form they do, wouldn't it make sense to model them around the most successful examples of such, maybe learn from the Finns[159], or learn from the Russian Shchetinin school[160]. Meanwhile though, in the absence of such innovative alternatives, give serious thought to home schooling[161] or unschooling[162]. Discover 55 serious reasons to homeschool[163], or, from a Christian perspective, if that's what floats your boat, 100 good reasons for how your child and the rest of your family, can benefit from the experience of homeschooling[164].

Countries and Borders

I have never considered myself by any means to be a patriot. I am not a nationalist. I do not consider myself to be English, nor Norwegian, nor Polish, nor Australian, although I might lay down claim to any of those. I might carry a passport, but resent being obliged to do so, and do so only because I know it has been my nature to travel and I am more than well aware of the neurotic bullying border guard officials, who unquestioningly follow orders of no real value; who would probably deport, detain or imprison me if I were to do otherwise. If I had more strength, I'd probably burn my passports publicly, as I have belief in the words of Gandhi that if a law is unjust it is our moral obligation to disobey it openly. My rather broad interpretation of "unjust" encompasses anything which opposes true spiritual values.

"To blame the poor for subsisting on welfare has no justice unless we are also willing to judge every rich member of society by how productive he or she is. Taken individual by individual, it is likely that there's more idleness and abuse of government favours among the economically privileged than among the ranks of the disadvantaged." - Norman Mailer

I do not believe in countries nor boundaries. It is my opinion we are, each and every one of us, aliens here. It just happens that geographically the region named England is the first country I visited, this time. But no territory belongs permanently to any one country. Boundaries cannot last as their divisions represent brute statements carved by military force. A time will come when there will be no politically imposed borders. "The Earth" will be our country, our home, and we will be forever aware that we are all just "visiting".

Humanity and all life on earth has already suffered enough due to politically imposed borders. I have to live somewhere and am happy of all places it is here, in Australia. But I do not belong here. I do not belong to any one country. All nationalism is in some way or another a form of fascism and as such, is a hindrance toward world peace. A danger to true progress. Nationalists are neurotic. Human history is ample proof of this.

One day, the goods of this earth will be distributed unselfishly according to the needs of all life. But equality cannot be established by force, it will come from the heart. Take our children, look in virtually every school throughout the world and you will see how openly "love of country" is taught, this generally sows the seed of misunderstanding and often even hatred toward other nations; this must and will change.

> ### Mango-Zen
>
> Sasho, the old Zen monk, is dying. News soon reaches all his worldly Sannyasins and they come running to pay their last respects.
>
> Rishiki, his most favoured pupil, hears of the imminence of the passing of his master. Quickly, he makes his way to the market.
>
> "But where do you go Rishiki!? Your master lies in the opposite direction!"
>
> Ignoring these words, he moves on to the market. There, he searches high and low and finally finds a single stall with a single Durian; Durio Graveolens. The last of a small out-of-season pile. A fruit he knows only too well his master has an especial fondness toward.
>
> Rishiki arrives at the dwelling of Sasho. Sasho turns to him and says, "Ahh, Rishiki, at last, you are here" - "Yes Master, the obvious is indeed always profound".
>
> They exchange smiles.
>
> Rishiki splits the ripe and ready durian and offers the opened fruit to his teacher.
>
> Seeing, the frailty and ebbing life-force of their master, one young student looks to him and says: "master. You are about to leave us. Please, if you could summarise all of your teachings into one brief sentence, what would it be?".
>
> "Ahh, little, Rimpo", the master sighs. He takes up the soft red flesh of the durian and places it on his tongue. Everyone waits.
>
> "This Durian is Excellent!" he smiles.
>
> At that, Sasho leaves us to continue his voyage in other realms.

Littering

While still on the subject of cleaning up, I'd like to point out how perfectly natural it is to litter. In our lost true environment, if we pick an orange from a tree, there is nothing wrong with pealing it and throwing the peel anywhere. It will quickly be broken down and absorbed by the earth becoming one with it. Fast forward to the 21st century though and that banana skin is more likely to be a sweet or lolly wrapper, plastic trash[165] or coke can. We fight our ingrained true nature each time we diligently search for an appropriate place to discard such. I am not suggesting we throw our wrappers just anywhere! I am merely pointing out how, because we have distanced ourself so much, there is a constant up hill struggle to keep that distance. Work, money, debt etc.

Flights

I reckon overweight passengers on board commercial flights should be charged for their extra weight. It strikes me as being unfair that I should be charged for taking a few extra kilos of luggage, when some people weigh more than my luggage and I combined. Not that I fly any more, it's been years. Just saying! I'm not implying that naturally taller people be charged more, just there should be some kind of chart comparing height with weight, and those on the plus side of a reasonable range, charged excess weight ticket fees.

Actually, governments should be offering us annual financial bonuses for staying healthy and slim!

"Privately owned banks create money out of nothing & loan it out at interest. All modern money is literally debt owed to them,. The economy is a casino, central banks control the game, and the house always wins!" - Brad Olsen

Money

Now, money's something we could talk of until the fat lady sings, the way it is so grossly unevenly distributed and the illusion of the banks and financial systems. Clearly, while it is still being used, something needs to be done to share the riches fairly. What would help is if somehow money could be made perishable, such that if a dollar doesn't change hands, it gradually depreciates in value. Yeah, I'm scratching my head on that one myself. I don't have it all clear in my head yet, but the idea doesn't seem completely infeasible. There should be a "maximum" wage, as well as a minimum one, maybe the maximum one could be just five or six times the minimum one.

Anything earned above that should either disappear completely, or be put toward some kind of fund whose goal is to help heal the world. I believe also it would be wise to stop inheritance, maybe not entirely, but certainly to an extent, such that the wealth in the hands of the rich families is slowly released. Certainly if anyone dies without an heir, leaving money in the bank, that money should not be swallowed by the bank, but contributed to the "heal the planet" fund. Yes, yes, I am aware of the complexity of all this, but this system of money is already mind bogglingly complex such that a few added rules would not be out of the question.

Taxes

Let us decide what should happen to tax money, if we wish to ensure no money is spent on arms and the military, we should be able to nominate more precisely how it is spent. It should be about "we, the people" and what we want, not what is decided for us.

Death

I believe it was Benjamin Franklin who once said "the only certain things in this world are taxes and death". I'd question his judgement there, but that's not what I'm here

> "Governments don't want well informed people, capable of critical thinking. That is against their interests. They want obedient workers, people who are just smart and indoctrinated enough to run their machines and do the paperwork. And just dumb enough to passively accept it." - George Carlin

for, however having given my tuppence worth on taxes, I'll throw in another tuppence on death. We should be allowed to take care of our own dead. I'm someone who isn't dying to get into a cemetery in the dead centre of a town somewhere, I'd like for someone to bury me in my garden and plant a fruit tree on top of me. The idea that my body must by law be buried in a casket, six feet under in a cemetery, or burnt otherwise to cinders, is a clear money making scam. Why waste precious wood just to put someone's body in! Cardboard should suffice and will help the corpse to break down quicker. Or just throw the body in a hole, cover with earth and plant tree!

Calendar

> What do you call a dinosaur with an extensive vocabulary? Thesaurus Rex.

A reform of the calendar. Starting the year on the northern hemisphere winter solstice. This would seem logical enough. There could be thirteen months with every month consisting of twenty eight days and starting on a Monday, (thus the first of every month would be Monday, and we would no longer have to remember how many days in each month) and New years day can be an extra day simply called "new years". Every leap year there can also be a "leap day" added to the end of each year. The month names can be rechristened, as they clearly make little sense as they now stand (Sept = 7? Oct=8? Nov=9? Dec=10?). This way calendars can be basically the same every year. Think how much paper is wasted from calendars that are printed and then discarded because they are not sold. Such a waste. This would not be the case if all years were the same. Americans could finally conform with the rest of the world and have their dates listed in the dd/mm/yy format!

Language

It seems a great idea to have an international language that is both one hundred percent logical and completely non biased to either gender or language group, simple, coherent and elegant. A language that has both room for ambiguity, but also can be completely clear with no room for confusion. The purpose of such a language could not only be a compulsory neutral language subject in all countries of the world, but also to be a main focus for all language translation. It amazes me that google and such, have people working to translate to and from every combination of known language, when it would be far simpler to have language translation purely in to, and out of this new proposed language, a hub language. With such a concentrated focus, translation progress would be increased manifold. Simplifying global communication greatly.

> "Kindness is a language which the deaf can hear and the blind can see."
> - Mark Twain

Several languages exist already that partially fulfil the criteria of such a language, Esperanto[166] being probably the most known and used of them, however, although it definitely has potential to be fine tuned it fails through being European language and gender biased. More recent attempts like lojban although quite logical leave no room for ambiguity; a necessity for successful translation from any language that is fundamentally ambiguous.

> I once did a theatrical performance about puns. It was a play on words.

For example, I wish the English language contained a neutral third person pronoun that wasn't "it". One that could be used instead of he and she to describe a living person or being where gender was unimportant. Needless to say, whenever I write he and refer not to a specific person, the real pronoun I mean is genderless.

Alternate Fuel

Mechanically minded I am NOT. I've heard rumours that Tesla[167] came up with some free energy source which could be transmitted wirelessly[168], and I'd definitely vote for that if it

"All people everywhere should have free energy sources.. Electric power is everywhere present, in unlimited quantities and can drive the world's machinery without the need for coal or gas" - Nikola Tesla

were vouched for as safe, authentic and no longer suppressed.

Meanwhile though, in the absence of such enlightened technology, I believe a simple, relatively eco-friendly solution for fuelling vehicles, could be quite easily obtained from water and sunlight. I would not myself know where to start, but nevertheless have enough knowledge to recognise this as quite readily doable. Basically it would involve solar roof panels for a free stationary power supply, this power could then work on extracting the hydrogen from water fed to it. The hydrogen could be channelled into high pressured tanks, which then in turn could be connected to a modified lowly combustion engine and used to fuel one's vehicle. All problems

"The greatest crimes in the world are not committed by people breaking the rules, but by people following the rules. It's people who follow orders that drop bombs and massacre villages" - Banksy

you might foresee with such an undertaking could be overcome. Fossil fuels could very quickly and efficiently become a thing of the past.

It seems pretty self evident to me, that we have this massive battery of energy called the sun that likely gives more energy in a single day than could possibly be needed to keep humans going for far more than an entire lifetime. So the question needs to be asked, what have all the real geniuses out there, already come up with, and what has been suppressed?

Modern day alternatives are impending environmental catastrophes. Whether it be inevitable oil spillage[169], or the even more destructive Chernobyls and Fukushimas (said to currently be spilling three hundred tonnes of radioactive waste into the ocean daily[170]). They are Pandora's boxes just waiting to be cracked open, and with each one that is, hope shines ever dimmer..

(Positive side note: Peru is reported to be offering free solar energy to the countries poorest inhabitants[171]. Bravo Peru!)

> Remember when all those kids got asthma from solar panel exhaust, toxic wind turbine ash got into your food, and clean energy contaminated the drinking water?.. Yeah, me neither!

Jobs

Over the course of the past couple of centuries, the percentage of population working in Primary industry has decreased manifold. The number now is at an all time low, with barely even 10% of the work force involved in food production. This ever lowering of primary industry percentage, is an ever increasing disaster. Everyone needs to re-evaluate the work line they have chosen as most jobs in today's world are clearly worthless. Indeed, many jobs are less than worthless and outright harmful to Gaia. This is something we all need to wake up to. This whole idea of all gainful employment being positive, and blatant unemployment being negative, when clearly neither is necessarily the case, needs to be rethunk.

Conspiracies

It's my opinion that the media often doesn't report the truth, and when it does do so, frequently only reports it partially. We are lied to so often, so cleverly, on such a large scale, that for many the lies are blatantly obvious and those with such insight will inherently distrust all printed and reported media filtered word. Especially anything to do with politics, the military, terrorism and health, most news of which, generally have much bigger stories and ulterior motives behind them. Yet, despite the blatant lies, there are still a large percentage of the populace who blindly buy into all reported words, trusting them unquestioningly and believing the conspiracy theorists to be nothing more than overly paranoid, tin-foil hat, crackpots. I believe the public is rarely ever made openly aware of the government's true agendas, and the true extent which money and power has corrupted the controlling elite.

Probably the biggest conspiracy out there concerns food, which has been transmogrified so much, it no longer bears semblance to anything that nature ever intended for us. All manner of addictive chemicals are added to hook long term customers and make them unwilling to even consider to reflect too much upon the subject. I know there are many people who as soon as the word "vegetarian" is mentioned, will express hatred toward it. The last thing they want to do is have their habits challenged! We need to learn to open our eyes, ears and hearts, and question everything. I've already said, I'm happy for you to challenge this book. I want everything challenged!

Music

Music is another powerful tool that can be used for good or evil. Soft, gentle, notes can sooth the soul and bring more peace into the world. Contrarily, harsh, chaotic music can do the opposite, increasing more suicidally chaotic thoughts. Especial concern needs to be taken to avoid "The Devil's interval[172]", a combination of notes said to be so dissonant that it makes one tense and restless, and often brings on a state of extreme negativity. That's not something any of us need!

> "We cannot tolerate or allow those who are undeservedly in power to deny the human race of attaining its true collective potential any longer." - Damien Carrion

The best music will be had in Eden, when the birds all sing in harmony with the gentle breeze, and brooks hum melodiously through our orchards, when the frogs and toads sing us their evening lullabies, and the mellifluous chorus of insects cantillate resonantly.

> *"And that is a story that no one can beat,*
> *When I say that I saw it on Mulberry Street."*
> **- Dr. Seuss**

EPILOGUE

Many great ideas start out as blasphemy and it's clear to me, the crux of what I'm talking of here will be seen by many as just that. Blasphemous hogwash! How dare I suggest that nature can be improved? Do I think I can do better than God? What right do I have to interfere with nature? I can already sense the accusations. I propose no interference though, in fact it is not so much about focusing on changing the

> Did you know there are roughly 1500 newspapers, 1100 magazines, 9000 radio stations, 1500 TV stations, 2400 publishers? All owned by only 6 corporations!

world, as changing oneself. I recognise if one places a focus on what's wrong, one can easily miss out on the ever present joys too. I know I've tried to point out the extent to which human society is mad, but beyond the realms of this book, my main focus is on what can be, in a lighter, more love filled world and on bringing my own world more into sync with such an eventuality.

I don't go around telling everyone how they should live, or tut tutting at their choices, in fact, there are many people in my social sphere who have no real idea of my life choices, as well as good friends and family who I know do not share all my view points, but we get on nevertheless. If people ask, I'm always happy to share and answer any questions and I try and always do so maintaining a sense of humour in the process. Hence the terribly corny jokes. I think it's important to be light hearted in the face of adversity and to not let the negativity of a demented world get the better of oneself.

I've not tried to claim the guidelines I've outlined are inflexible fact. I don't *know* that they are. If you think this is a cop out and that I'm avoiding responsibility, then you have things twisted, As stated in the disclaimer, I am not responsible for you or your concluded

> "Being a good person doesn't depend on your religion, your race, your skin colour or culture. It depends on how good your heart is, and how well you treat others." - Unknown

thoughts. Each of us alone has responsibility for the decisions and choices we make and the conclusions we reach. Whether or not someone else thought of them first is irrelevant. I have reached my conclusions and they have proved successful with me. I am confident with what I am saying, but at the end of the day, each must find their own confidence!

I'm not saying anyone has to live their lives any given way, only stating how I chose to live mine and how I chose to see mine progressing and yes, how I believe the world would be better off, if others followed suit.

I have also not tried to claim, that by us all eating just fruit, we would automatically solve all the world's problems. It should be clear, many things must change before even the fruit we eat is ideal, and thus Eden compatible. However, the potential for it to be such, is clearly present and with time, focus and effort, can become just that; Eden compatible.

> "There are some people who could hear you speak a thousand words and still not understand you. And there are others who will understand without you speaking a word." - Unknown

Although I have no doubt some will determine I am judging others for their actions, I acknowledge it is not my place to do so. My ribbing at 801010 and Doug Graham are light hearted, and not meant to offend anyone, I acknowledge that there are well meaning people following his path, many very aware of the circle of compassion and the need for it to blossom. Let it be known that the judgement I pass is on actions themselves and not on he or she committing those actions. Although, in retrospect, I guess this is a slight cop out, because clearly I am judging. I'm ruling humankind, especially the Homer-sapiens, and all life on earth to be suffering an affliction of insanity. Don't worry about my judgement though, in and of itself it is without consequence. I suggest you settle on your own equally inconsequential conclusions.

I can't stress this enough, I know you may think of me as an incredibly critical person, but my basic philosophy is really that we should all do what we *truly* believe is correct, so if you think this book is all nonsense, and wholeheartedly believe shod omnivorism is what this world is all about, and the path you believe wisest to remain on, then that is precisely where I believe you should remain. However, IF you feel offended by my critic and judgement, but are unable to state clearly why, then I suspect there may be a deeper reason.

> "Talk about your blessings, more than you talk about your problems" - Unknown

Probably cognitive dissonance. I mean why should you care what I think? If you're confident with your beliefs why should you feel threatened or offended by mine? If anything, feel pity for me. I don't care, because I'm confident with my beliefs.

If there are questions which I've forgotten to tackle, and issues I've neglected to address and I'm sure there are, try and take a step backwards and answer them yourselves. If you're wondering where honey lies in my food tower and you truly grok what I'm saying, surely you can find a place for it. I'm hoping that Eden Fruitarianism is not just another concept that gets embraced by people who can't think clearly and who end up dragging it through the mud.

Yes, Eden Fruitarianism may be radical. But to heal and transform the planet, radical changes are needed; until radical becomes the new normal!

From the profound and gloomy depths of shod omnivorism, it might seem like Eden Fruitarianism is purely an emotional choice, however, the higher one eats on the proposed food tower, the more blatantly clear it becomes, just how much it is truly a logical choice. So if you are reading this book a hundred years from now and nothing appears to have improved, you can rest assured, the spirit of what I write is still very much alive. It is immortal and has been around since time immemorial, I have tasted from its source, and it is still as fresh and pure as ever, forever flowing, infinitely waiting for us all to join in.

ABOUT ME

Most people *believe* they *know* things, I believe my self professed wisdom comes from *knowing* I *believe* things. I see a profound difference between the two outlooks. I concede that my knowledge is limited and recognise I don't have all the answers. None of us do, none of us

> I see no good reason to act my age.

are perfect, least of all myself, (and I speak from profound personal experience!). Recognising such failings though, should not prevent us from moving forward. Our ignorance and inability to see the road ahead with perfect vision and clarity, should never prevent us from trying to improve ourselves.

Let me very briefly introduce myself. Born in 1961, I call myself Mango and together with my life partner, Kvĕta, live a peaceful life in the tropics of FNQ Australia. You might think, it's all well and good that I write of these things from my comfortable life of relative abundance, but that for most people things aren't so

> I'm currently also reading a book about anti-gravity. I can't put it down.

straight forward, with far too many difficulties and obstacles impeding one's progress and journey. This would be quite an unfair assessment though. I too started out life as an unwitting, zombie flesh eating, shod omnivore, in a large town (Wellingborough) in the grey, damp drabness of Northamptonshire, England. As a young teenager I began plotting my escape, and in 1982, the day before my 21st birthday, I fled England's shores. I've since lived in other large towns and cities, in countries with winters longer than summers, I've faced many daunting challenges throughout my journey, and impatiently yearned for the life I have now, evoking divine powers of manifestation to bring it slowly toward me. I've been impatient and frustrated when things haven't always been smooth, and the journey has not been short either, but taken many years, indeed, decades. But each time I have experienced a revelation, I have never lost sight of its significance, and strived to ever live

> "Never waste your time trying to explain who you are, to people who are committed to misunderstanding you."
> - Unknown

life more in fulfilment of such revelations. One must take on the attitude that abundance is more something we tune in to, rather than something that requires blood, sweat, tears and the almighty($) dollar.

The first half of my autobiography is now complete, it explains more of myself and my life and revelations, my hardships and joys and narrow escapes throughout that journey. The second half, Volume Two, will likely not be completed until sometime in 2020 or later. I will announce on my website[173], blog[174] and Facebook page[175] once it is finally available.

This book is also available in Italian[176], Serbian[177], Spanish[178], and the Czech language[179]. Other language translations are also in the pipeline, so please check my Spotlight page at Lulu[180] to see what languages are available, both as Ebooks and printed books.

Books by Mango

Destination Eden[181]
(Eden Fruitarianism Explained)
(Uncommon Sense – Volume 1 of 4)

The Eden Fruitarian Guidebook[182]
(Uncommon Sense – Volume 2 of 4)

2020 Vision[183]
(Veganism++)
(Uncommon Sense – Volume 3 of 4)

Topsy-Turvy World[184]
(Uncommon Sense – Volume 4 of 4)

Discovering Eden Fruitarianism
An Autobiography - Volume one[185]
(Awakening to Veganism)

Arnold Trevor Cirrus[186]
(Goes to the Congo)
(An Illustrated Book for Kids)

REFERENCES

1　"Pure Fruit", Vimeo Video, 1:01:44, documentary about Mango & Květa, by Emile Bokaer, 2012, https://vimeo.com/36666602

2　"Quite Possibly the most Eye Opening Six Minutes Ever on Film", Video, 06:15, August 16, 2013, https://www.minds.com/blog/view/201538/quite-possibly-the-most-eye-opening-six-minutes-ever-on-flm

3　Dr. Seuss, "The Lorax", Book

4　Catharine R Gale, "Research into IQ in childhood and vegetarianism in adulthood: 1970 British cohort study", the BMJ, 28 October, 2006, http://www.bmj.com/content/334/7587/245

5　Virginia Messina, "Empathy, intelligence and the vegetarian brain", *examiner.com*, June 1, 2010, http://www.examiner.com/article/empathy-intelligence-and-the-vegetarian-brain

6　Marc Bekof, "Brain Scans Show Vegetarians and Vegans Are More Empathic than Omnivores", *Psychology Today*, July 12, 2012, https://www.psychologytoday.com/blog/evolved-primate/201005/empathy-is-what-really-sets-vegetarians-apart-least-neurologically-speak

7　"Cognitive Dissonance", *Wikipedia*, Accessed June 24, 2015, https://en.wikipedia.org/wiki/Cognitive_dissonance

8　"Abattoir worker slits puppy's throat because he couldn't afford vet's bill", *Daily Mail Australia*, December 9, 2011, http://www.dailymail.co.uk/news/article-2071775/How-Abattoir-worker-slit-puppys-throat-aford-vets-bill.html#comments

9　"Brazilian Pork Sausage Piglet Prank", *YouTube video*, November 29, 2012, https://www.youtube.com/watch?v=NG4WhppBNCM

10　Unknown Author, "Vegetarians live longer and have better health," *Eating Ecologically*, Accessed June 24, 2012, http://www.eateco.org/Medical/Vegetarian.htm

11　Ashley Capps, "Catching Up With Science: Burying the 'Humans Need Meat' Argument", *Free From Harm*, July 17, 2013, http://freefromharm.org/health-nutrition/catching-up-with-science-burying-the-humans-need-meat-argument/

12　Helen Stockebrand, "Comparative Anatomy Chart," *photobucket*, Accessed June 25, 2015, http://s39.photobucket.com/user/orange-light/media/debates/comparison.jpg.html
　　Michael Bluejay, "Humans are naturally plant-eaters," *Vegetarian Guide*, Updated October 2014, http://michaelbluejay.com/veg/natural.html
　　Wishro, "Science Verifes that Humans are Frugivores," *Scribd*, July 5, 2009, http://www.scribd.com/doc/17111888/Science-Verifes-Tat-Humans-Are-Frugivores

13　George Dvorsky, "Prominent scientists sign declaration that animals have conscious awareness, just like us," *io9*, August 23, 2012, http://io9.com/5937356/prominent-scientists-sign-declaration-that-animals-have-conscious-awareness-just-like-us

14　Alastair Bland, "From Pets to Plates: Why More People are eating Guinea Pigs,

The Salt, April 2, 2013,
http://www.npr.org/sections/thesalt/2013/03/12/174105739/from-pets-to-plates-why-more-people-are-eating-guinea-pigs

15 Stevo, "Video Facts of meat production," *meatvideo.com*, Accessed June 25, 2015, http://www.meatvideo.com

16 Gary Youofsky, "Best Speech You Will Ever Hear," *YouTube* video, December 22, 2010, https://www.youtube.com/watch?v=es6U00LMmC4

17 Sheeplecorporation, "The Earthlings video", *YouTube* video, April 17, 2011, https://www.youtube.com/watch?v=19eBAfUFK3E

18 Keith Akers, "Animal Brothers, 4th Letter," *compassionatespirit.com*, Accessed June 25, 2015, http://www.compassionatespirit.com/animal_brothers_4.htm

19 Mark Hawthorne, "The Mental Health Consequences of Killing For a Living," *Occupyforanimals*, March/April 2011, http://occupyforanimals.wix.com/meat#!slaughterhouse-workers/czcf

20 Chris Winter, "The Case for Vegetarianism, Explained by a child" *YouTube video*, June 4, 2013, https://www.youtube.com/watch?v=sJNntUXyWvw
Conufan, "Adorable Irish Girl Explains Why She doesn't want to eat meat," *YouTube video*, July 5, 2015, https://www.youtube.com/watch?v=mMgJYQgYS24

21 Free The Slaves, "Slavery is Everywhere," *freetheslaves.net*, Accessed June 26, 2015, http://www.freetheslaves.net/about-slavery/slavery-today

22 Doris Lin, "How Many Animals are Killed Each Year?", *animalrights.about.com*, Accessed June 26, 2015, http://animalrights.about.com/od/animalrights101/tp/How-Many-Animals-Are-Killed.htm

23 "Slaughterhouses", *Wikipedia*, Last Modifed June 16, 2015, https://en.wikipedia.org/wiki/Slaughterhouse

24 Noam Mohr, "Animal Death Count in US," *animaldeathcount*, Accessed June 26, 2015, http://animaldeathcount.webnode.com/all-animals-2011/

25 ADAPTT, "Real time Kill counter," *ADAPTT*, Accessed June 26, 2015, http://www.adaptt.org/killcounter.html

26 Isha Datar, "Why your burger should be grown in a lab," *CNN report*, August 9, 2013, http://edition.cnn.com/2013/08/08/opinion/datar-lab-burger/index.html?hpt=hp_c4
Laura June, "Your Meat Addiction is Destroying the Planet," *The Verge*, August 13, 2013, http://www.theverge.com/2013/8/13/4605528/your-meat-addiction-is-destroying-the-planet-but-we-can-fx-it

27 Kaita Moskvitch, "Modern Meadow aims to print raw meat using bioprinter," *BBC News*, January 21, 2013, http://www.bbc.co.uk/news/technology-20972018
Ryan Whitman, "3D Printed meat could soon be cheap and tasty enough to win you over," *GEEK News*, February 12, 2013, http://www.geek.com/news/3d-printed-meat-could-soon-be-cheap-and-tasty-enough-to-win-you-over-1539410/

28 Edward Immel, "Evolution of the words vegetarian and vegan," *Gentle World*, July 28, 2012, http://gentleworld.org/whats-in-a-word/

29 Irish Vegetarian Society, "Vegetarian and Vegan Defnitions," *Vegetarian Society of Ireland*, January 25, 2014, http://www.vegetarian.ie/defnitions

30 Sara Talyor, "The Benefts of extended breastfeeding," *The Daily Mom*, May 16,

2016 2013, http://dailymom.com/nurture/the-surprising-benefts-of-extended-breastfeeding/

31 Animals Australia, "Dairy Cows Fact Sheet," *Animals Australia the voice for animals*, Accessed June 26, 2015, http://www.animalsaustralia.org/factsheets/dairy_cows.php

32 VM Sathish, "AL Ain 'Super Cow' gives100 litres of milk a day," *Emirates247*, June 21, 2011, http://www.emirates247.com/al-ain-super-cow-gives-100-litres-of-milk-a-day-2011-06-21-1.403953

33 Voiceless, "Australia Battery Hen facts," *Voiceless – The Animal Protection Institute*, Accessed June 26, 2015, https://www.voiceless.org.au/the-issues/battery-hens

34 Unknown, "Facts about caged egg-laying hens," *nocagedeggs.com*, Accessed June 26, 2015, http://nocagedeggs.com/caged-eggs.htm

35 Amy Remeikis, "'Free range eggs' defnition scrambled, *The Brisbane Times*, July 29, 2013, http://www.brisbanetimes.com.au/queensland/free-range-eggs-defnition-scrambled-20130728-2qshq.html

36 Animals Australia, "The Truth about cows, dairy and leather," *Animals Australia Unleashed*, Accessed June 26, 2015, http://www.unleashed.org.au/animals/cows.php

37 Vegan Mainstream, "A Fur Farm Experience," *vegan Mainstream*, Accessed June 26, 2015, http://www.veganmainstream.com/2011/11/30/vegan-means-being-a-voice-for-animals-a-fur-farm-experience/

38 The Vegetarian Resource Group, "Why don't vegans use leather, silk or wool?," *The Vegetarian Resource Group*, Accessed June 26, 2015, http://www.vrg.org/teen/leather_silk_wool.php

39 Emily Moran Barwick, "Is Wool Vegan? Is it humane?," *Bite Size Vegan*, Accessed 26 June, 2015, http://www.bitesizevegan.com/ethics-and-morality/is-wool-vegan-is-it-humane

40 Vegan Peace, "Wool Facts," *Vegan Peace*, Accessed June 26, 2015, http://www.veganpeace.com/animal_cruelty/wool.htm

41 Christine Wells, "Why Vegans Don't Use –Silk," *Gentle World*, December 1, 2012, http://gentleworld.org/do-vegans-use-silk/

42 Mercy for our Sentients, "I am scared and don't want to die," *YouTube video*, May 29, 2009, https://www.youtube.com/watch?v=LUkHkyy4uqw

43 Left by the side of the hive, the bees will feed from the bucket.

44 "Marital Rape," *Wikipedia*, Accessed 26, June 2015, https://en.wikipedia.org/wiki/Marital_rape

45 "The Simpsons," *Wikipedia*, Accessed June 26, 2015, https://en.wikipedia.org/wiki/The_Simpson

46 Jong Gao, "Boys' urine-soaked eggs listed as local speciality, intangible cultural heritage," *The Ministry of Tofu*, March 11, 2011, http://www.ministryofofu.com/2011/03/boy-urine-soaked-eggs-listed-as-local-specialty-intangible-cultural-heritage

47 Chirs Pirillo, "Chocolate Covered Grasshoppers," *YouTube video*, 5:12, Uploaded June 30, 2009, https://www.youtube.com/watch?v=_qJ7TLwPbh0&feature=youtu.b

48 "The Grossest food You're Eating Every Day," *WorldTruth.TV*, Accessed June

27, 2015, http://worldtruth.tv/grossest-food-youre-eating-every-day

49 "Statistics for Chronic Disease," Australian Institute of Health and Welfare, Accessed June 27, 2015, http://www.aihw.gov.au/statistics-for-chronic-disease/

50 Fast Food – Exposing the Truth," *Cancer Council NSW*, February 22, 2013, http://www.cancercouncil.com.au/wp-content/uploads/2013/02/Fast-Food-Exposing-the-Truth-22-February-2013.pdf

51 "Chemotherapy Doesn't Work 97% of the Time - Dr. Glidden," *GreenMed TV*, April 7, 2013, http://tv.greenmedinfo.com/chemotherapy-doesnt-work-97-of-the-time-video/

52 Christine Luisa, "Exposing the fraud and mythology of conventional cancer treatments", October 12, 2011, http://www.naturalnews.com/033847_chemotherapy_cancer_treatments.htm

53 Arjun Waila, "Man With Stage 3 Colon Cancer Refuses Chemotherapy and Cures Himself With Vegan Diet," *Collective Evolution*, July 21, 2013, http://www.collective-evolution.com/2013/07/21/man-with-stage-3-colon-cancer-refuses-chemotherapy-cures-himself-with-vegan-diet/

54 Herbert M. Shelton, "The Hygienic System Vol III - Fasting and Sunbathing," 3rd Revised Edition, 1950, http://www.soilandhealth.org/02/0201hyglibcat/020127shelton.III/020127.toc.htm

55 Morris Krok, "Fruit, the food and medicine for man", Book

56 Edmond Szkely, "The Essene Science of Fasting and the Art of Sobriety: Guide to Regeneration in Health and Disease", Book

57 "Douceur et Harmonie: Domain Mamn Terre," *Douceur et Harmonie*, Accessed June 25, 2015, https://douceurharmonie.wordpress.com/
"Douceur et Harmonie," *Ecovillage Networking*, Accessed June 25, 2015, http://sites.ecovillage.org/douceur-et-harmonie-domain-maman-t

58 Arnold Ehret, "Mucusless Diet Healing System" (see pages 16,-18)
Arnold Ehret, "Rational Fasting", Book

59 "Vegan Diet impacts California Prison," Vegetarian Spotlight, January 9, 2011, http://vegetarianspotlight.com/2011/vegan-diet-impacts-california-prison/
"Saved By A Vegan Prison," *Vegetarian Spotlight*, December 20, 2012, http://vegetarianspotlight.com/2012/saved-by-a-vegan-prison/

60 Emanuel Barling Jr, Esq and Ashley F. Brooks, RN, BSN, "Medical Doctors Have Little or No Knowledge of Nutrition," *howtoeliminatepain.com*, June 9, 2011, http://howtoeliminatepain.com/medical-doctors-have-little-or-no-knowledge-of-nutrition-because-medical-schools-ofer-little-or-no-education-on-nutrition-vitamins-or-minerals

61 Kelly M Adams, "Status of nutrition education in medical schools," *NCBI*, June 18, 2008, http://www.ncbi.nlm.nih.gov/pmc/articles/PMC2430660/?tool=pubmed

62 Ben Goldacre, "What Doctors don't know about the drugs they prescribe", *Ted Talks*, June 2012, https://www.youtube.com/watch?v=RKmxL8VYy0M

63 Sarah C. Corriher, "Death Rates Drop When Doctors Go on Strike," *The Health Wyze Report*, Accessed June 27, 2015, http://healthwyze.org/index.php/component/content/article/502-death-rates-drop-when-doctors-go-on-strike.html

64 "Anopsology", *Wikipedia*, Accessed June 27, 2015, https://en.wikipedia.org/wiki/Anopsology

65 "Guy-Claude Burger", *Wikipedia*, Accessed June 29, 2015, https://fr.wikipedia.org/wiki/Guy-Claude_Burger (in French)

66 Loren Cordain, Ph.D, "The Paleo Diet," *The Paleo Diet*, Accessed June 29, 2015, http://thepaleodiet.com/

67 Mark Sisson, "Primal Blueprint 101", *Mark's Daily Apple*, Accessed June 29, 2015, http://www.marksdailyapple.com/primal-blueprint-101/

68 Dr. Douglas Graham, "Home of The 80/10/10 Diet and Dr. Douglas N Graham", *FoodNSport.com*, Accessed June 29, 2015, http://foodnsport.com/index.php

69 Douglas Graham, "The 80/10/10 Diet", Book

70 "Seed dispersal methods", *Wikipedia*, Accessed June 29, 2015, https://en.wikipedia.org/wiki/Seed_dispersal

71 Scott Zona, "Plants that use Ballistic seed dispersal", *Fairchild Tropical Botanic Garden*, Accessed June 29. 2015, http://www.virtualherbarium.org/gardenviews/GoingBallistic.html

72 Christopher Bird & Peter Tompkins, "The Secret Life of Plants", Book

73 "Mythbusters – Plants have feelings(primary perception)", *YouTube video*, Published October 16, 2012, https://www.youtube.com/watch?v=fStmk7e9lJo

74 "MythBusters", *Wikipedia*, Accessed June 29, 2015, https://en.wikipedia.org/wiki/MythBusters

75 "Secret Life of Plants and Telepathy", *YouTube video*, Uploaded August 22, 2010, https://www.youtube.com/watch?v=MPpURDTTf8k

76 "The Secret Life of Plants –Full", *YouTube video*, Published on October 9, 2012, https://www.youtube.com/watch?v=sGl4btrsiHk

77 Tafne Laylin, "New Study Shows Plants Talk to Each Other Trough the Soil", *inhabitat.com*, May 23, 2014, http://inhabitat.com/plants-talk-to-each-other-through-a-messenger-in-the-soil

78 R. Jenness, "The Composition of Human Milk", *NCBI*, July, 1979, http://www.ncbi.nlm.nih.gov/pubmed/392766

79 "World Class Bodybuilder is RAW VEGAN", *YouTube video*, Published July 3, 2012, https://www.youtube.com/watch?v=2dM1iU5e33k

80 "Vegans Bodybuilders dominate Mainstream Competition", *Vegan Bodybuilding & Fitness*, July 27, 2013, http://www.veganbodybuilding.com/?page=article_robert_austin_2013

81 "The China Study", *Wikipedia*, Accessed June 29, 2015, https://en.wikipedia.org/wiki/The_China_Study_%28book%29

82 Ross Horne, "The Health Revolution", Book

83 Sophie Egan, "Making the Case for Eating Fruit", *The New York Times*, July 31, 2013, http://well.blogs.nytimes.com/2013/07/31/making-the-case-for-eating-fruit/?_r=2

84 Derek Henry, "How to heal cavities naturally", *Live Free Naturally*, November 2013, http://livefreelivenatural.com/heal-cavities-naturally

85 "The Ayurvedic Doshas", *Wikipedia*, Accessed June 29, 2015, https://en.wikipedia.org/wiki/Dosha

86 Peter J . D'Adamo, "Eat Right For Your Type", Book

87 "Food Pyramid (Nutrition)", *Wikipedia*, Accessed June 29, 2015,

https://en.wikipedia.org/wiki/Food_pyramid_%28nutrition%29
88 "Water facts and fgures", IFAD, http://www.ifad.org/english/water/key.htm
89 "Livestock's Long Shadow", *Wikipedia*, Accessed June 29, 2015,
    https://en.wikipedia.org/wiki/Livestock%27s_Long_Shadow
90 Kate Good, "How Animal Agriculture Is Draining the World of Biodiversity",
    One Green Planet, September 29, 2014,
    http://www.onegreenplanet.org/animalsandnature/how-animal-agriculture-is-
    draining-the-world-of-biodiversity
91 Tamar Haspel, "Monocrops: They're a problem, but farmers aren't the ones who
    can solve it", *The Washington Post*, May 9, 2014,
    http://www.washingtonpost.com/lifestyle/food/monocrops-theyre-a-problem-
    but-farmers-arent-the-ones-who-can-solve-it/2014/05/09/8bfc186e-d6f8-11e3-
    8a78-8fe50322a72c_story.html
92 Michael Bloch, "Leather and Envionmental Issues", *Green Living Tips*, August
    24, 2012, http://www.greenlivingtips.com/articles/leather-and-the-
    environment.html
93 OneGreenPlanet.org, "Facts on Animal Farming and the Environment", *One
    Green Planet*, November 21, 2012,
    http://www.onegreenplanet.org/animalsandnature/facts-on-animal-farming-and-
    the-environment/
94 "Eating up the World: The Environmental Consequences of Human Food
    Choices," *livekind*, Accessed April 24, 2016,
    http://www.livekind.com.au/downloads/EUTW.pdf
95 "The Commonwealth Scientific and Industrial Research Organisation", *CSIRO*,
    Accessed June 29, 2015, http://www.csiro.au/
96 "Deep-Sea Fish STOCKS" *Eur-Lex Access to European Law*, Accessed June 29,
    2015, http://eur-lex.europa.eu/legal-content/EN/TXT/?uri=URISERV:l66053
97 "Shopping for fish? Why there's a catch", *The Sydney Morning Herald*, July 22,
    2013, http://www.smh.com.au/lifestyle/diet-and-fitness/chew-on-this/shopping-
    for-fish-why-theres-a-catch-20130722-2qdqi.html
98 "ISPM 15 - International Standards For Phytosanitary Measures No. 15",
    Wikipedia, Accessed Jun 29, 2013, https://en.wikipedia.org/wiki/ISPM_15
99 "Barefoot", *Wikipedia*, Accessed June 29, 2015,
    https://en.wikipedia.org/wiki/Barefoot
100 Mark Pagel, Walter Bodmer, "A Naked Ape Would Have Fewer Parasites", *The
    Royal Society*, August 7, 2003,
    http://rspb.royalsocietypublishing.org/content/270/Suppl_1/S11
101 Marilyn D. Story, "Personal and Professional Perspectives on Social Nudism",
    JSTOR, Accessed June 29, 2015, http://www.jstor.org/stable/3812606
102 Mark Storey, "Children, Social Nudity And Scholarly Study", *o2binsxm.com*,
    Accessed June 29, 2015, http://o2binsxm.com/childrenandsocialnudity.htm
103 "A comparison of pro- and anti-nudity college students on acceptance of self and
    of culturally diverse others", *NCBI*, September 2008,
    http://www.ncbi.nlm.nih.gov/pubmed/18686157
104 Mike Adams, "Sunscreen Causes Cancer", *Natural News*, May 29, 2008,
    http://www.naturalnews.com/023317.html AND
    Herbert Shelton, "The Health Benefits of Sunlight",

251

healingcancernaturally.com, Accessed April 24, 2016, http://www.healingcancernaturally.com/healingwithlight5.html#fastingandsunbathing

105 "Chaetophobia", *Wikipedia*, Accessed June 30, 2015, https://en.wikipedia.org/wiki/Chaetophobia

106 "Pogonophobia", *The Free Dictionary*, Accessed June 30, 2015, http://www.thefreedictionary.com/pogonophobia

107 "The Truth About Hair and Why Native Americans Would Keep Their Hair Long", *Science of the Spirit*, September 08, 2011, http://www.sott.net/article/234783-Te-Truth-About-Hair-and-Why-Indians-Would-Keep-Teir-Hair-Long

108 Mark, "45 Uses for Lemons", *ALTDrudge.com*, August 17, 2013, http://altdrudge.com/45-uses-for-lemons-that-will-knock-your-socks-off

109 "Here's What it Looks Like When you Don't Wash of your Makeup For a Month", *The Hufngton Post*, September 17, 2013, http://www.hufngtonpost.com/2013/09/16/makeup-premature-aging-_n_3936828.html?utm_hp_ref=mostpopular.

110 Visala Kantamneni, "These 8 Countries Have Banned Wild Animals in Circuses", *One Green Planet*, March 19, 2014, http://www.onegreenplanet.org/animalsandnature/10-countries-that-have-banned-wild-animals-in-circuses

111 Tafne Laylin, "Costa Rica is Closing its Zoos and Freeing All Captive Animals", *Inhabitat*, August 9, 2013, http://inhabitat.com/costa-rica-is-closing-its-zoos-and-freeing-all-captive-animals/

112 Laura Beck, "Vegan Dogs", *The Bark*, November 16, 2010, http://thebark.com/content/vegan-dogs

113 Chuck Raasch, "Cats kill up to 3.7 billion birds annually", *USA Today*, January 30, 2013, http://www.usatoday.com/story/news/nation/2013/01/29/cats-wild-birds-mammals-study/1873871/

114 "Paro Terapeutic Robots", *PARO*, Accessed Jun 30, 2015, http://www.parorobots.com

115 Jackson Landers, "Does your pets food contain dead pets?", *Slate*, April 19, 2013, http://www.slate.com/articles/health_and_science/science/2013/04/what_is_in_pet_food_zoo_animals_sick_livestock_dogs_and_cats_from_shelters.single.html

116 Nicole Adams, "Radoslaw Czerkawski to be held on bail – Read the Comments", *examiner.com*, December 19,2013, http://www.examiner.com/article/radoslaw-czerkawski-to-be-held-on-no-bail-puppy-doe-will-see-justice

117 Dave Munger, "Up to Half of All Humans Are Infected by a Cat-Borne Parasite", *Seed Magazine*, Accessed June 30, 2015, http://seedmagazine.com/content/article/toxic_house_cats

118 "Worldwide Pet Overpopulation Epidemic", *Dog Breed Info Center*, Accessed June 30, 2015, http://www.dogbreedinfo.com/articles/breedersvsrescues.htm

119 "Animal Overpopulation", *Oxford-Lafayette Humane Society*, Accessed June 30, 2015, http://www.oxfordpets.com/index.php?option=com_content&view=article&id=61

120 Otto Spijkers, "Understanding Bokito the Gorilla", *The Netherlands School of Human Rights Research*, May 21, 2007, http://invisiblecollege.weblog.leidenuniv.nl/2007/05/21/understanding-bokito-the-gorilla-that-es

121 "Brumby", *Wikipedia*, Accessed June 30, 2015, https://en.wikipedia.org/wiki/Brumby

122 "The Golden Rule", *Wikipedia*, Accessed June 30, 2015, https://en.wikipedia.org/wiki/Golden_Rule

123 Daniel Burke, "The World's Fastest Growing Religion is...", *CNN*, April 4, 2015, http://edition.cnn.com/2015/04/02/living/pew-study-religion

124 "The Lioness and The Oryx", *BBC News*, January 7, 2002, http://news.bbc.co.uk/2/hi/africa/1746828.stm

125 Rivlin, "True Story – Vegetarian Lioness", *Youtube Video*, Accessed April 24, 2016, https://www.youtube.com/watch?v=eI1kcyKx1yQ

126 "Tikkun Olam", *Wikipedia*, Accessed June 30, 2015, https://en.wikipedia.org/wiki/Tikkun_olam

127 Abby Miller, "Good Deeds, Not Belief in Christ, Required for Salvation Says New Pope", *Addicting Info*, May 23, 2013, http://www.addictinginfo.org/2013/05/23/good-deeds-not-belief-in-christ-required-for-salvation-says-new-pope

128 "Natural Law Party", *Wikipedia*, Accessed June 30, 2015, https://en.wikipedia.org/wiki/Natural_Law_Party

129 Steven Bancarz, "Studies Reveal Group Meditation Can Lower Crime Rates, Suicide Rates, and Car Accidents in Surrounding Cities", *Spirit Science and Metaphysics*, Accessed June 30, 2015, http://www.spiritscienceandmetaphysics.com/studies-reveal-group-meditation-can-lower-crime-rates/

130 "Goldilocks Zone", *Rational Wiki*, Accessed June 30, 2015, http://rationalwiki.org/wiki/Goldilocks_Zone

131 "Axial Tilt", *Wikipedia*, Accessed June 30, 2015, https://en.wikipedia.org/wiki/Axial_til

132 "Walkabout," Wikipedia, Accessed June 30, 2015, https://en.wikipedia.org/wiki/Walkabout

133 "Witchetty Grub", *Wikipedia*, Accessed June 30, 2015, https://en.wikipedia.org/wiki/Witchetty_grub

134 "Permaculture" *Wikipedia*, Accessed June 30, 2015, https://en.wikipedia.org/wiki/Permaculture

135 "Vegan Organic Gardening", *Wikipedia*, Accessed June 30, 2015, https://en.wikipedia.org/wiki/Vegan_organic_gardening

136 Clare Leschin-Hoar, "It's Not a Fairytale: Seattle to Build Nation's First Food Forest", *TakePart*, February 21, 2012, http://www.takepart.com/article/2012/02/21/its-not-fairytale-seattle-build-nations-frst-food-forest

137 Masanobu Fukuoka, "The One-Straw Revolution", Book

138 Ann Jones, "Men of the Trees - Richard St. Barbe Baker interview", *ABC – RN*, August 26, 2012, http://www.abc.net.au/radionational/programs/ofrack/men-of-the-trees/4188212

139 Ashley Capps, "12 Reasons You May Never Want to Eat Turkey Again", *Free from Harm*, November 7, 2013, http://freefromharm.org/animal-cruelty-investigation/12-reasons-you-may-never-want-eat-turkey-again/

140 John 16:21, Romans 8:22

141 Richard Stone, "Who are the Illuminati", *Red Ice Creations*, Accessed July 1, 2015, http://www.redicecreations.com/specialreports/whoilluminati.html

142 Stephen Lendman, "The true Story of the Bilderberger Group, and What they May be Planning", *Global Research*, June 1, 2009, http://www.globalresearch.ca/the-true-story-of-the-bilderberg-group-and-what-they-may-be-planning-now/13808

143 "Trilateral Commission: World Shadow Government", *Illuminato News*, Accessed July 1, 2015, http://www.illuminati-news.com/trilateral-commission.htm

144 Alcohol and Public Health: Alcohol-Related Disease Impact (ARDI), Centers for Disease Control and Prevention, Accessed July 1, 2015, http://nccd.cdc.gov/DPH_ARDI/default/default.aspx

145 Robert Gable, "The Toxicity of Recreational Drugs", *American Scientist*, Accessed July 1, 2015, http://www.americanscientist.org/issues/pub/the-toxicity-of-recreational-drugs/99999

146 "Merck drug company vaccines admits injecting cancer viruses", *Live Leak*, November 17, 2007, http://www.liveleak.com/view?i=327_1195303011

147 "Vaccines did not Save us – 2 centuries of Ofcial Statistics", *Child Health Safety*, Accessed July 1, 2015, https://childhealthsafety.wordpress.com/graphs

148 Andrew Baker, "The Vaccine Hoax is Over. Documents from UK reveal 30 years of cover-up", *nsnbc internatinal,* May 10, 2013, http://nsnbc.me/2013/05/10/the-vaccine-hoax-is-over-freedom-of-information-act-documents-from-uk-reveal-30-years-of-coverup/

149 Dave Mihalovic, "You want to vaccinate my child? No problem, just sign this form", *Prevent Disease*, August 9, 2013, http://preventdisease.com/news/13/080913_You-Want-To-Vaccinate-My-Child-No-Problem-Just-Sign-This-Form.shtml AND "Physician's Warranty of Vaccine Safety", *Prevent Disease*, Accessed August 15, 2015, http://preventdisease.com/pdf/Warranty-of-Vaccine-Safety-English.pdf

150 Lorena Nessi, "Scared of the Sun – The Global Pandemic of Vitamin D Defciency", Brain Blogger, June 16, 2013, http://brainblogger.com/2013/06/16/scared-of-the-sun-the-global-pandemic-of-vitamin-d-defciency

151 "MythBusters - Plants have Feelings, Primary Perception", *YouTube video*, Published October 16, 2012, https://www.youtube.com/watch?v=fStmk7e9lJo

152 Dean Nelson, "Man claims to have had no food or drink for 70 years", *The Telegraph*, April 28, 2010

153 "Hilton Hotema", *Wikipedia*, Accessed July 1, 2015, https://en.wikipedia.org/wiki/Hilton_Hotema

154 Hilton Hotema, "Man's Higher Consciousness", Book

155 "Sungazing", *Wikipedia*, Accessed July 1, 2015, https://en.wikipedia.org/wiki/Sungazing

156 Vinny Pinto, "Sungazing - Observations and notes from a veteran Sungazer",

Sungazing, September 23, 2007, http://sungazing.vpinf.com/
157 "Peace Pilgrim", *Wikipedia*, Accessed July 1, 2015,
https://en.wikipedia.org/wiki/Peace_Pilgrim AND
"Peace Pilgrim", *Peace Pilgrim - Official Website*, Accessed July 1 2015,
http://www.peacepilgrim.org
158 Boyan Slat, "How the Oceans can clean themselves", *YouTube video*, Accessed
July 2, 2015, https://www.youtube.com/watch?v=ROW9F-
c0kIQ&feature=youtube_gdata_playe
159 Olga Khazan, "The secret to Finland's Success with Schools", *The Atlantic*, July
11, 2013, http://www.theatlantic.com/international/archive/2013/07/the-secret-
to-fnlands-success-with-schools-moms-kids-and-everything/277699
160 "Mikhail Petrovich Shchetinin - Kin's School - Lycee School at Tekos", *David
Icke*, March 28, 2009, http://www.davidicke.com/forum/showthread.php?
t=59310
161 Liesl Den, "11-year old shares her thoughts about homeschooling.",
Parents.com, March 4, 2014,
http://www.parents.com/blogs/homeschool-den/2014/03/04/homeschool-den/11-
year-old-shares-her-thoughts-about-homeschooling/
162 "Unschooling", *Wikipedia*, Accessed April 24, 2016,
https://en.wikipedia.org/wiki/Unschooling
163 Stefanie Relfe B.Sc., "55 Serious Reasons Why You Should Homeschool",
relfe.com, March 9, 2014, http://www.relfe.com/wp/children/55-serious-reasons-
homeschool/
164 Marianne Sunderland, "100 Reasons Why Homeschooling is Good for
Families", *Abundant Living*, December 8, 2014,
http://www.mariannesunderland.com/2014/12/08/why-homeschooling-good/
165 "This Film Should be Seen by Everyone" *Why Don't you try this?*, November
21, 2013, http://www.whydontyoutrythis.com/2013/11/this-flm-should-be-seen-
by-the-entire-world.html
166 "Esperanto", *Wikipedia*, Accessed July 2, 2015,
https://en.wikipedia.org/wiki/Esperanto
167 "Nikola Tesla", *Wikipedia*, Accessed July 2, 2015,
https://en.wikipedia.org/wiki/Nikola_Tesla
168 "Discover How to Use a 100 Year old Device to Generate Free Electricity",
Nikola Tesla Secret, Accessed July 2, 2015, http://www.nikolateslasecret.com/
"Nikola Tesla", *Free Energy*, Accessed July 2, 2015,
http://free-energy.ws/nikola-tesla
169 Laura Moss, "The 13 largest oil spills in history", *Mother Nature Network*, July
16, 2010, http://www.mnn.com/earth-matters/wilderness-resources/stories/the-
13-largest-oil-spills-in-history AND
"Montara Oil Spill", *Wikipedia*, Accessed July 2, 2015,
https://en.wikipedia.org/wiki/Montara_oil_spill
170 Mike Adams, "Fukushima leaking 300 tonnes of radioactive water daily",
Natural News, August 13, 2013,
http://www.naturalnews.com/041610_Fukushima_radioactive_leak_state_of_em
ergency.html AND
Gary Stamper, "Your days of eating pacific fsh are over", *Collapsing into*

Consciousness, Accessed July 2, 2015, http://www.collapsingintoconsciousness.com/at-the-very-least-your-days-of-eating-pacifc-ocean-fsh-are-over

171 Timon Singh, "Peru to Provide Free Solar Power to its 2 Million Poorest Citizens", *Inhabitat*, July 23, 2013, http://inhabitat.com/peru-solar-power-program-aims-to-give-electricity-to-the-countrys-2-million-poorest-citizens/

172 Finlo Rohrer, "The Devil's Music", *BBC News*, April 28, 2006, http://news.bbc.co.uk/2/hi/uk_news/magazine/4952646.stm

173 Mango Wodzak, "Mango's Website", *fruitnut.net*, Accessed March 2, 2013, http://www.fruitnut.net

174 Mango Wodzak, "Mango The Raw Vegan Fruitarian", *Mango's Blog*, Accessed March 2, 2013, http://mangodurian.blogspot.com.au/

175 "Mango Wodzak on Facebook", *Facebook*, Accessed March 2, 2013, https://www.facebook.com/mangodurian

176 Mango Wodzak, "Destinazione Eden", *Impronte Di Luce*, Accessed April 25, 2016, http://www.improntediluce.it/schede_libri/destinazione_eden.html

177 Mango Wodzak, "ODREDIŠTE RAJ", *esotheria.com*, Accessed April 25, 2016, http://esotheria.com/shop/zdrav-zivot-telesni-hram/odrediste-raj/

178 Mango Wodzak, "Destino Eden", *lulu.com*, Accessed April 25, 2016, http://www.lulu.com/content/paperback-book/destino-ed%c3%89n---bolsillo/18476740

179 Mango Wodzak, "CÍL RÁJ", *lulu.com*, Accessed April 25, 2016, http://www.lulu.com/shop/mango-wodzak/c%C3%ADl-r%C3%A1j-bro%C5%BEovan%C3%BD/paperback/product-22593033.html

180 "Mango Wodzak – Author Spotlight", *lulu.com*, Accessed April 25, 2016, http://www.lulu.com/spotlight/DestinationEden

181 Mango Wodzak, "Destination Eden – Eden Fruitarianism Explained", *FruitNut*, Accessed September 30th, 2020, http://fruitnut.net/destination-eden

182 Mango Wodzak, "The Eden Fruitarian Guidebook", *FruitNut,* Accessed September 30th 2020, http://fruitnut.net/the-guidebook

183 Mango Wodzak, "2020 Vision - Veganism++", *FruitNut*, Accessed September 30th 2020, http://fruitnut.net/2020-vision

184 Mango Wodzak, "Topsy-Turvy World", *FruitNut*, Accessed October 1st, 2020, http://fruitnut.net/topsy-turvy-world

185 Mango Wodzak, "Discovering Eden Fruitarianism – Volume One", *FruitNut,* Accessed September 30th 2020, http://fruitnut.net/autobiography

186 Mango Wodzak, "Arnold Trevor Cirrus", *FruitNut*, Accessed September 30th, 2020, http://fruitnut.net/arnold-trevor-cirrus

Printed in Great Britain
by Amazon

32499609R00146